"The wisdom in this book i[s] sometimes in life all we need [is] we're not alone on this journey all the contributing writers as they teach us the lessons they've learned along the way, and feel uplifted with the knowledge I have gained through their stories."

- **Mena Suvari** (Actress - *American Beauty, American Pie*)

"A buffet of both practicalities and inspiration. Whether you dip in for something specific, or read it cover-to-cover, you'll find something here that you can put to immediate use."

- **Jane Espenson** (Writer/Producer - *Once Upon A Time, Buffy the Vampire Slayer, Husbands*)

"The timing is perfect for a book such as this with some of the most informative and inspirational blogs out there. Helenna has an uncanny sense of bringing together the most talented ladies."

- **Marci Liroff** (Casting Director - *Mean Girls, Footloose, E.T.*)

"In a day and age where gender equality is popping up in the news on a regular basis, *Ms. In The Biz* is the 'one small step for women, one giant leap for womankind' that is desperately needed in the entertainment industry."

- **Eric England** (Writer/Director – *Contracted, Madison County*)

"The industry has changed, most excuses we have for not pursuing our dreams come down to one thing - fear. The fear of starting being the worst offender because it leads to fear of finishing, and the fear of failure. This extremely useful collection of articles and real world tips helps us push through the never ending battle with ourselves, so we can get to work creating."

- **Evan Glodell** (Director - *Bellflower)*

"I wish this book had been around when I was getting started, it is full of invaluable advice and loads of inspiration…it will save you from pitfalls and help you find your way in this strange world that is Hollywood."

- **Patrick Gallagher** (Actor - *Night at the Museum, Glee, True Blood*)

"Beginner or veteran - overwhelmed or clueless - this is some realistic advice from different perspectives to help you stay sane and feel a little less lonely."

- **Lynn Chen** (Actress- *Saving Face*, Food Blogger - *The Actor's Diet*)

"*Ms. In The Biz* offers one of the greatest gifts mentors and a supportive community can offer all of us at any level of our careers: realistic expectations. That's not to mean stifling or dimming your hopes or dreams - nor hyping or indulging your pipe dreams - but rather offering clarity on just what could possibly be achieved from here, now - and how. Success leaves clues. Here are some breadcrumbs to follow."

- **Heather Hale** (Producer, Writer, Director)

"Hollywood is changing fast. To survive and thrive, you need crystal clear goals, a game plan and the guts to keep going when things get tough. Luckily for you, *Ms. In The Biz* provides a road map that gets you from where you are now to where you want to go. I highly recommend this book."

- **Jason Brubaker** (Film Distribution Strategist – *FilmmakingStuff.com*)

"With our every choice, we are creating the Hollywood we want to be a part of. Helenna has built a community of leaders in our glorious industry and their voices beautifully align to inform, motivate, and inspire in this exciting new book."

- **Bonnie Gillespie** (Author, Casting Director, Coach)

"I love this book! I have been getting the *Ms. In the Biz* emails for a while now and this book is a lovely compilation of the best of those articles! I am all about positive energy and pursuing your dreams, and so is this book! I highly recommend you read this book. Wonderful tips to help you navigate this tricky entertainment industry!"

- **Denise Gossett** (Actress - *Get the Gringo, The Office*, Founder and Director of the *Shriekfest* Film Festival)

"Thriving in Hollywood! Tenacious Tales and Tactics from Ms. In The Biz is a must-read compilation for any woman navigating the current film entertainment industry. This tome of touching, revealing, and wise advice from working women in front of and behind the camera lets the rest of us know we're not alone - that other women are out there, looking out for us, and sharing their experiences with us so we can learn and succeed."

  - **Heidi Honeycutt** (Film Journalist, Festival Programmer)

"I devoured this book in one sitting. It feels like going to coffee with a group of your best friends while they talk shop. These new girlfriends of yours happen to be successful women who have been there and done that. You will walk away feeling like you know these women, as they impart their candid advice and help you set reasonable expectations. They will inspire you, not by some fluffy positive intention stuff, but by giving you real life tools and tactics to put your goals on track for success. A must read by anyone who wants real and practical advice on how to put your best foot forward in *The Biz*."

  - **Bridget Jurgens** (Managing Director of Dog & Pony, a movie poster design agency)

"This book's refreshingly positive and *relatable take* on how to thrive in Hollywood serves as validation that success is a soul thing. It's actionable; and the product of an open mind and a broadened perception on how to get ahead. Helenna's brand of wisdom will inspire women and show them how to catch their dreams instead of *just* chase after them!"

  - **Nicole Taylor Roberts** (Cannes Nominated Filmmaker and Head of RocketLight Films)

"This book is a Godsend."

  - **Madeline Brewer** (Actress - *Orange is the New Black, Hemlock Grove*)

Thriving in Hollywood!

Tenacious Tales and Tactics

from

Ms. In The Biz

compiled by

Helenna Santos

and

Alexandra Boylan

msinthebiz.com

Dedicated to all of the families and friends who support artists.

Thank you. We love you.

And to:

Bobbie Muralt, Ruben Santos, Helen Muralt, and Barry W. Levy

Miriam and William Boylan, and John K.D. Graham.

You help us fly.

Table of Contents

PART THREE: The Practical and The Tactical

PART FOUR: Don't Hate, Collaborate!

PART FIVE: Conquering "The Biz"

PART SIX: Recharge and Take Charge

Introduction

I am completely and utterly addicted to sharing information. When I find something cool, no matter what it is, I want to get that knowledge out into the world as quickly as possible so that other people can rock out with me. In the spring of 2013, I knew I had a serious itch to scratch when I found myself constantly wanting to share what I'd learned while pursuing a career in the entertainment industry. In fact, I was pretty sure that a lot of the women I knew in the business would be hungry to share things as well. I also had a hunch that there would be many women yearning to connect with other like-minded ladies who were also walking down this gorgeous yellow brick road.

Msinthebiz.com came about with the sole purpose of taking what I had learned so far in the entertainment industry, along with the knowledge of over a hundred other awesome ladies, and delivering that over the interwebs in order to help people navigate through the often murky waters of show business. I wanted to create a home for growth, positive community and entrepreneurial spirit that appealed to women in all areas of the business. I wanted to cultivate a big roundtable of knowledge where we could all jam together and thrive.

Entertainment is a tricky industry that operates like no other business on earth, and many people start out thinking that things are going to be much easier than they actually are. This journey is a long one, and I truly believe that it's all about the steps we take that make up our career as a whole. So for me, *Ms. In The Biz* has always been about showing not only the awesome glitz and glamour of the spotlight, but also the daily elbow grease that is required along the way.

When *Ms. In The Biz* writer Alexandra Boylan came to me and said she wanted to help me put together a compilation book, I jumped at the chance to share some of the key articles that have been published on *msinthebiz.com* in our first year. All of these articles have great information to help not only those new to the business, but also veterans looking for proof that they aren't alone on this epic journey.

Whether you are a "Ms." in the biz, or a Mister supporting all your industry sisters, my hope is that you'll find you are not alone on this path, and that after reading these tenacious tales and tactics, you'll be well on your way to THRIVING.

Helenna Santos
Actor/Producer/Writer/Founder of Ms. In The Biz

***

As fast as the technology age is changing, so is the entertainment industry. By the time you have mastered something—BOOM—there is something new to understand. Being an artist now means you must also be a businessperson, and there really is no way around that. Whether you are an actor, makeup artist or a cinematographer, you now have to consider yourself under the broader title of "filmmaker". To truly grasp this industry and take charge of your career, you must first embrace and understand the WHOLE picture. This book is exciting because it gives advice, knowledge and stories from different aspects of the film industry that everyone can take something away from. We are all working together to create ART, like all of the colors coming together to create an image on a blank canvas.

The greatest gift we can posses is the knowledge passed down by the ones who have gone before us. Learning and being willing to listen is our greatest ally. Instead of living in jealousy or judgment, if we sit in a place of learning, we can grow to greater heights than we could ever imagine. And that is what this book will give you, the wisdom and armor to defeat, conquer and thrive in a business that has no problem knocking you down as hard as it can. You have chosen a challenging career path, but inspiration is the key to never giving up. Allow these pages to inspire you and drive you forward to live the life you have always dreamed of. Be ready to take on the challenges ahead with advice from those who have been where you want to go.

Alexandra Boylan
Producer/Writer/Actress

ACKNOWLEDGMENTS

There are so many people who were instrumental in getting *msinthebiz.com* off the ground. It's impossible to mention everyone since a big reason that the site has flourished is because of the many readers all over the globe, but I'll do my best to remember all of the people without whom I could never have done this. So here goes…

To those that helped me when I was building the site and had absolutely no idea where to start, THANK YOU. Nic Baisley, Verona Blue, Jeff Turner, Kristen Nedopak, Brianne Grebil, Zain Meghji, Amber Krzys, and Marie Forleo and B School, you all rock my world.

To Angelique Toschi, the site's Social Media Coordinator, and Holly Elissa Dignard, who acted as Associate Editor in the early stages of the site, I could not have been able to wrap my head around the enormity of this site without you both.

To Jordan Mizell (aka Saint Pepsi) whose awesome cartoon artwork of me lives and breathes in her black dress and bangs, you are AMAZING!

To Rachel Schmidt for her fantastic editorial skills, and Susan Lee and Alissa Juvan for their proofreading eyes, THANK YOU!

To all of the companies and people who have supported the site from the beginning:
Taylor McPartland and Darren Marble from *FilmBreak*, my brother in social media mania Brian Rodda from *Brian Rodda Consulting*, my sister in entrepreneurship and one of my greatest supporters and besties for life Leah Cevoli, my dear friend and confidant Jackie Fogel whom I am so honored to have in my life and her incredible husband Jeremy Fogel, Marc Royce of *Marc Royce Photography*, Risdon Roberts, Dani Lennon, and Alex Santori because you are all awesome, Verona Blue from *CodeBloo*, Lynn Chen and *The Actor's Diet*, *FilmSnobbery*, Bonnie Gillespie and the *Self Management for Actors* team, Jason Brubaker of

Filmmaking Stuff fame, *Nedopak Productions' The Geekie Awards*, Trevor Algatt and AJ Meijer from the *Inside Acting Podcast*, Gedaly Guberek the *Awesome Web Guy*, David H. Lawrence XVII with *Rehearsal the App*, Blair Hickey and Brian Wold of *Casting About*, and Adam and Sylvia Hendershott of *The Headshot Truck*, and my symbiotic sister Alyssa Swanzey.

To my family and friends who have supported me in all of my artistic endeavors, especially my mother Roberta Muralt, father Ruben Santos, grandmother Helen Muralt, and my husband Barry W. Levy: I love you all very much. And to my amazing siblings Grace Chin, Rose Tom, Ed Santos, and Julius Santos, along with the rest of the Santos family, the Muralt/Maloff family, and Sharon McGowan who is practically family, you have all been such an amazing support to me and I thank you deeply from the bottom of my heart. This book exists because you have always believed in me.

To my Canadian gals: singing soul sister and "women in boots" partner Rhosyln Jones, gorgeous survivor and beautiful yogi Rachel Schmidt, strong and sexy thespian momma Sasa Brown, and the magician with a camera and a Buddha baby Sara Borck - you + me + two bucks. You will always be some of my #1 ladies. Thank you for your friendship and unending belief in me. And to my "LA Mother" Barbara Deutsch: a million THANK YOU's.

To the many teachers that I have had over all of these years, thank you for sharing your brilliance and passion with me. Hopefully this book and the *Ms. In The Biz* website help to bring a piece of knowledge and light to the world in the same way your wisdom has affected me.

And finally, the site and this book wouldn't exist without all of the incredible writers who have contributed their incredible articles. Because I have new writers joining the site each month, as of the date this went to print, those amazing women are: Alana Husband, Alex Santori, Alexandra Boylan, Alexis McDonough, Allison Vanore, Ally Zonsius, Alta DeKoven, Amber Plaster, Amber Sweet, America Young, Anastasia Washington, Andrea Adams, Andrea Vicunia, Angelique Toschi, Annie Wood, April Audia, Ashleigh Nichols,

Ashley Wallace, Aubrey Arnason, Brittany Carson, Barbara Deutsch, Brea Grant, Briana Hansen, Brianne Grebil, Candy Washington, Carrie Certa, Cat Doughty, Catherine Kresge, Celia Aurora de Blas, Chrissy Lynn, Christine Moore and *Crafty Shodmanship Productions*, Cindy Marie Jenkins, Cindy Sciacca, Cooper Harris, Crix Lee, Crystal Chappell, Dallas Travers, Dana Waldie, Dani Lennon, Dani Morales, Deanie Mills, Deborah Smith, Elisa Teague, Emily Grace, Erika Diehl, Erin Brown, Erin Henriques, Etta Devine, Fanny Veliz, Georgina Ware, Hadley Meares, Hayley Derryberry, Heather Olt and Dellany Peace, Heidi Honeycutt, Holly Elissa Dignard, Holly L. Derr, Jackie Fogel, Jacqueline Steiger, Jane Jameston, Jen Levin, Jennifer Ewing, Jennifer Gullick, Jessica Leigh Smith, Joline Baylis, Julia Camara, Kat Castaneda, Kate Hackett, Katherine Di Marino, Katrina Hill, Katt Shea, Kim D'Eon, Kristy Spraggon, Kosha Patel, Kris Evans, Krishna Devine, Kristen Nedopak, Kristyne Fetsic, Kylie Sparks, Leah Cevoli, Lee Hulme, Leesa Dean, Linda Antwi, Lindsay Cooley, Lissette Schuster, Lizza Monet Morales, Maayan Schneider, Madeline Merritt, Malia Miglino, Marilyn Anne Michaels, Misty Madden, Musme Bravo, Nami Scott, Natasha Younge, Nicole Larson, Nicole Mandujano, Patty Jean Robinson, Paula Rhodes, Rachel Levine, Rhoslyn Jones, Rhym Guisse, Robin Bain, Robin Phelps, Sallyanne Ryan, Samara Bay, Sandra Seeling, Sarah Louise Lilley, Shamia Casiano, Shanice Kamminga, Shannon Bowen, Silvana Gargione, Siobhan Doherty, Stacey Anne Shevlin, Stephanie Kaliner, Stephanie Piche, Stephanie Pressman, Stephanie Thorpe, Susan Rubin, Sylvia Hendershott, Tamara Krinsky, Tanya Ihnen, Tara Platt, Taryn O'Neill, Teresa Jusino, Tisha Rivera, Trina Vargas, Tristen MacDonald, Verona Blue, Vicky Ayala, Victoria Marie, Violeta Meyners, and Wendy Braun.

And finally to Alexandra Boylan: without your help this book would not exist. You constantly inspire and challenge me to achieve more than I think I can. You are a dream partner. I can't wait to work with you on more projects in the future.

And to all of the ladies and gents who are out there every single day making their way through this crazy industry of ours, your journeys inspire me every single day. THANK YOU.

Helenna Santos

PART ONE: Begin It

Choose Yourself
By Barbara Deutsch

Game over. You win. If you choose you. How long can a truly creative person wait to be "picked" before she tears her hair out, punches a wall, or eats so much frozen yogurt she gains 10 pounds while convincing herself "it's not ice cream"? A very long time. We can tough it out as long as Mickey Rourke did in *The Wrestler*. Who invented waiting for permission to have a kick-ass career? Nobody. It's a lie that has been passed around for so long. Actually, in the old days, and I'm talking 60's, 70's, even the early 80's, there was a dance of artistry being in sync with the business. There were three or four people called back for an audition, a couple of people making decisions on a script, directors directing a whole season, book publishers publishing books without having a marketing plan or buzz in advance, and singers and bands getting a record deal without "playing out" for years.

Yes, those days were different from today, but today what's possible is that if you don't wait for someone to give you permission to be spectacular, you can be seen by the whole freakin' world. The only way I know how to guide people is to first have them surrender to their gifts. Meaning, if you want desperately to be a screenwriter, director, actor, producer, fine artist, and it's becoming a tough road, there may be other areas that you excel in and the door to that may be open a bit wider at the moment. DO NOT BE AFRAID to go there. I promise you, you will not lose your dream. In fact, if you take your hand off that dream wheel for a bit, and it could be a moment, a week, a month, it may need some fresh space and air anyway. Give it a breather. Surrender and play in another arena. Long ago if you took your hands off the wheel you would be considered a flake. Now if you don't for a moment, you could end up lonely and poor. (Too

3

dramatic? I guess.) Stop blaming "them." Go to the door that's inviting you in. Look for it. It's there.

Choose to jump. Don't wait for someone to agree with your choice. Who cares? What people think of you and your desires is none of your business. Stop defending yourself. Just play fully in whatever you want. It is such a service to your soul, not to mention that you will make a difference in the world, which is, I'm sure, what you wanted in the very beginning of the dream anyway. If you can't get on a series, make one. If you can't sell your screenplay, film it yourself. Or do a short that has a teeny budget. Do something that has a beginning, middle and an end and feel accomplished. My friend Pete plays guitar. He will NEVER be out of work. He can play in a band, a show, someone's living room or the street. Passion. It's passion and freedom. It's choosing YOU.

***

Barbara Deutsch is the creator of the *Barbara Deutsch Approach*, a unique teaching and coaching concept for people in the film and television industry. As a successful acting teacher and coach, Barbara knows about dreams, the rewards of their pursuit, and the sorrows of feeling stuck. Bringing over 25 years of experience to the table, she works with those in front of the camera and behind the scenes, acting as a Personal Champion and consultant.

How to Get Out of Your Own Way and Start Kicking Ass
By Madeline Merritt

One of the hardest things to do in life is to get out of your own way. You:

a) Have big dreams, but don't have a manageable checklist.

b) Want to accomplish big things, but don't know where to start.

c) Want to expand creatively by developing a new skill, but are afraid of being a beginner.

d) Sit at home feeling paralyzed because of your massive to-do list.

e) Hate yourself for not living up to your potential, and you think others are judging you for that as well.

And this cycle of self-loathing COULD continue on indefinitely…

But it won't. Not anymore. Not after today. ***Today, you have decided to begin the process of changing your life, upping your creativity and working towards goals that will fulfill you.*** That is because today, you are embracing who you are in the present and where you would like to be in the future. You are beginning the process with a great big liberating hallelujah of **ACCEPTANCE**.

A lot of us have dreams and goals that are massive: they seem un-doable in their current "ginormous" state, so we stare at them, wasting time, and not getting any closer to fulfilling our potential or our skillsets. Let's say we do need new skills to get the job done: well, it's hard to mobilize to learn the skills we need to achieve our dreams when we are sitting in a place of doubt and inertia.

Are you one of these people? Well, I am.

Let me tell you about my dreams in this biz: I am passionate about storytelling. I am in this industry because I love to tell stories that entertain, inspire, and bring new perspectives to people from different backgrounds to facilitate understanding and compassion. Thus far on the plinko board we call Hollywood, I have pursued this endeavor through acting, thinking that if I had a platform, I could make a difference. I am tired of this old model: I want to be a creator, not just someone that communicates other people's ideas. I love acting and I want to up my game career-wise, while also pursuing my own creative endeavors and collaborations.

The lack of material for strong young women like myself can be quite disheartening. There are also many other reasons, including the way women on-screen are portrayed, that I dream of a day where I am not just in front of the camera but writing, producing, and even directing my own projects.

The problem is: I am stuck. I am in my own way, and that is frustrating as hell. As much as I want to step up as a leader and organizer, someone that gets projects off the ground, I am still in that place where I am a do-er in that second tier sense. While I can commit and contribute to projects, and some of my ongoing relationships are manifesting themselves in new opportunities, *I am not at the helm of my own biz destiny.*

Like many of you, I am trying to improve myself, my strategy, my opportunities, and my performances, all the while juggling a job that keeps a roof over my head, a smartphone, and enough funds to attend necessary networking events, workshops, and acting classes. Whew.

While I don't feel I've led the most organized career in the world, after nearly four years in Los Angeles, I feel I am really getting somewhere, and so it is time to step up my game. NOW.

Here is my four-part plan to getting out of my own way, starting TODAY! (And you can do this too!)

1) Acknowledge where I have room to grow. Let go of the shame and admit it!

I have a list of Industry "duhs" and "dreams" that I haven't been keeping up with. They are my blocks. You probably have some too.

2) Honor the things I have done right so far.

You do this too! Write down all the awesome things you *have* achieved.

3) Pledge to abandon Bad Habits (one or two) for a set period of time (e.g. 30 days).

I am a procrastinator. The bad habits I developed in college (which included lots of cramming in the library around finals week and pulling off excellent grades) don't work as well in a life that doesn't often give you deadlines or finals. This industry is a marathon.

Procrastination has been my drug of choice, and I'm ready to set my goal, starting today, to eliminate two things from my life for the next 30 days.

4) Make short-term goals for the month to fill up this new free time.

Make reasonable, doable goals and see how many you can check off in that month, with all your new free time.

I am ready, I have goals in sight, and I am taking a pledge to let go of some of my bad habits so I can move forward professionally and artistically, because I have found ACCEPTANCE with where I am at and where I want to go.

Now what can you accomplish in the next 30 days if you take the PLEDGE???

Once you accept where you are in the present, it frees you to remove those stuck blocks and achieve the dreams in your heart.

Happy accepting!

***

7

Part actress, part writer, part producer and director, **Madeline Merritt** believes in telling stories that connect us to each other and remind us of our own humanity. She lives to entertain: from bold comedic performances to thoughtful dramatic characters, Madeline is a consummate chameleon who is able to bring diverse roles to life. With a long history of experience in front of and behind the camera, she brings practical know-how, diverse skills, and a spirit of optimism to all of her projects and working relationships. She is inspired by women leaders in entertainment and is a supporter of equality for women in media and the greater world.

When You Believe It, So Will We
By Georgina Ware

Five years ago when my husband left his nine-to-five job for the ability to work for himself, I think I silently panicked for what felt like, well, forever. Although I knew it was a smart move to quit his job because— creatively—it was a crime that he wasn't out there sharing his talents with the world, the *illusion* of the security that his survival job brought our family made me second-guess his decision. It would fascinate and simultaneously irritate me to watch how his immense confidence in his ability to succeed never faltered. While I could be found in the corner counting to ten, wondering how certain bills were going to be paid trying not to internally combust, he remained calm in his conviction that we were always going to be taken care of. I have to admit, I envied his control and belief that he was already a success with or without clientele knocking at his door.

At the start of his business, when clients were nonexistent, he still conducted himself as though he ran a million dollar corporation. He never cut corners, he never treated anyone differently regardless of if they were a paying customer or someone who was bartering services with him, and he always went above and beyond in regards to customer service. It didn't take long before word got out about his exceptional talent, and paying clients were lining up to photograph with him.

One evening we were sitting out back, and I asked him what his secret was and how he knew that he was going to make it. He just smiled, and in a calm voice said, "I didn't." My shocked look had him howling in laughter and he decided to elaborate. He proceeded to explain that for once in his career, he was at a place where he was doing what he *wanted* to do rather than what he needed to do. It wasn't that he was now a name brand in the industry, nor that he was making millions—it was much simpler than that. He was just doing what he loved.

He chose to no longer come from a place of need, which, if you're not careful, can turn into desperation. He understood that there was never any guarantee of financial success, but the personal satisfaction in doing what he was meant to do was worth the gamble. If he wanted others to believe in his brand, his talents, and what he had to offer, then he needed to be the first person to wholeheartedly believe in them too. He realized that when he was photographing he was in his sweet spot. That there was no other profession out there that made him feel more exhilarated, more alive, and more at purpose in knowing that his photographic creative eye was making a positive difference for other people. And that became his driving force. He truly came from the angle that **when you do what you love, that in itself is the truest gift**; the money that follows is just the added blessing that someone appreciates your worth. Even though logically he understood he needed to work to help provide for our family, he chose to make a simple shift in his thinking and understanding: that it is far healthier to come from a place of love rather than a place of need.

In the days that followed, our conversation had me thinking. How many people go into business with the wrong intention? I think we've all been approached by a pushy salesperson who was desperate to sell us something they didn't believe in or that we didn't need. Either we cave in and buy what they are selling (just to get them to go away) or we get angry and slam the door. What about the actor that goes into auditions or meetings with agents or managers from a place of desperation? I completely understand that burning desire to sign with an agent you really want or to book that great paying role. But when you allow desperation to settle into your bones, you stunt your ability to let the true essence of who you are to authentically shine through. When you can learn to separate the need to succeed versus the simple *want* and desire to do what you love, you open up the doors for so much more abundance and opportunity to come your way.

I found this poem on the wall in my husband's photo studio and it made me smile:

> *"They say for every light on Broadway there is a broken heart, an unrealized dream. And that's the same in any profession. So you have to want it more than anyone else, and you have to be your own champion, be your own superstar, blaze your own path, say yes to opportunity, follow your instincts, be eager, and passionate, keep learning, nurture your real and lasting relationships, don't be a jerk, and free your imagination so you can become all that you want to be."*
> – Sutton Foster

Over the years, unbeknownst to me, my husband was teaching me this very simple, yet valuable, lesson. When he decided to open his own photography business, he chose to be his own champion blazing his own path, all while doing it from a place of love.

My wish is that you all find that sweet spot in your personal journey through this crazy world we love called show business.

***

Georgina Ware is a writer, health coach, and showbiz mom to three living in LA. She enjoys helping other parents (and adult actors) learn the business of acting without losing their minds. Along with her husband, she co-owns *Kevin Michael Photography*, an LA based headshot and portrait photography studio. When she's not busy assisting with large photo shoots, managing acting careers, or doing freelance design or writing jobs, you will find Georgina helping others live a healthier and happy lifestyle through her business as an Independent Distributor for *It Works! Global*.

Are You Too Busy To Create Art?
By Kristen Nedopak

There are two types of people in this business: artists, and those who make believe they are creating art but are too caught up in the hustle of it all to let the divine force of creativity leak in.

Ouch. It's true though, isn't it? I don't mean to say hard work isn't what's needed in the world of entertainment. It is. Tenfold. What I am saying is that the longer we work in this industry (especially if we feel we have not achieved "success"), the more we get wrapped up in the hustle, in being "busy" with too many things to do and places to be. And then we sometimes neglect the reason we came here in the first place: to create art.

I partially blame it on a city that spits out far more rejection than it does validation, regardless of talent. How can the vulnerability needed to create art survive when our spirits are neglected so often? With so many facets to cover: publicity, social media, tech, training (the list is too huge to include it all), we are spread too thin to focus on what really matters. We find ourselves wounded, with little time and energy to do what we love, so we turn to mindless things like making sure every email in our inbox is read and responded to. That makes us feel as if we've accomplished something that day.

Over the last few years, I found myself in the busy body camp and I can tell you one thing for certain: it's a death trap for the spirit. How do we know if this trap has taken hold? Ask yourself: are you on an incredible body high after a long day of work? Do you come home with more energy than you left with and you can't stop talking about how amazing your day was? Or are you exhausted, frustrated, too tired to think straight, angry, and maybe a little depressed? Or do you feel guilty that the work you did wasn't what you wanted to do today?

Here's the thing: following your heart will never lead to any of that crap. You *should* be on a high. If you're not, it's time to make changes.

To stay creative, we must allow ourselves time to simply be—enough time to clear the clutter from our brains and let inspiration take hold. That's where creativity lies.

Here are four things that get me back into my artist self:

1) Don't let the world in until you're ready.
TIME! Where did it go? There is never enough of it! *We need more time!* This is why most of us sleep next to our phones. Email, texts, social media sites—they are the last thing we see before sleeping, and the first thing we see when we wake up. We have this concept in our heads that we must be productive 24/7 because everyone is waiting on us. Ok, but how productive can you truly be in a state of constant chaos? When does your brain get a break to recharge?

The best advice I've ever taken came from my former career coach Kristine Oller, who had one rule: every day she'd make time for herself before she "let the world in". It was *Kristine's* time to do whatever she wished—whether it be write, read or pour her soul into making a delicious breakfast—before she even considered opening email or dealing with *someone else's* needs. Truth is, we all need alone time to be at peace with our inner selves, to recharge and regroup, so we can be in the right mindset to tackle our insanely busy schedules. Even if it's just five minutes to close your eyes and breathe, it's *you* time.

When I give myself alone time, I feel my mind is calm and at peace. I'm even more productive because I can think straight and my decisions are made by instinct, not forced, overworked thoughts. I am able to make a clear distinction between pointless busy work and tasks I need to do to move forward, and the day feels lighter. I have the power to say no to requests that don't feed my soul (thank you, instincts), and I don't feel one bit guilty about it. Best of all, I find myself being more creative.

2) Remember the good times.

I remember being quite the hippie art student, filled with creativity, covered in paint, wearing homemade clothes that looked more like costumes than fashion. I'd stay up all night listening to music, painting, drawing, dancing (yes, by myself). My hair was ratted and up in some effortless, fun 'do. I loved nature and was forever traveling to new places to explore unknown landscapes, cultures, and people. I was enjoying life and, in turn, creating incredibly satisfying art.

So many inspiring elements were present back then, yet when I look at my life today, I'm void of almost all of them. I spend more time sitting at my computer than I do enjoying life around me. Very recently (literally this morning), I made a decision to pull those elements back into my life. I'll sit outside on my patio for an hour (or however long I want) before I begin my workday, to enjoy my nature-filled backyard. I bought a tribal drum on a recent trip to Hawaii, and I plan to play it each night. I'll get back into dancing and put more heart into cooking my meals—two things that put me in a very pleasant meditational state. I'll put tech away more often and enjoy the company of friends—in person (gasp!). I've gone as far as to plan a month-long trip to Hawaii this fall, where I'll stay in a tiny cabin on the cliff and write.

In short, I'll do things I know will put me in the same mindset as times past because, though life and responsibilities have changed, the things that charge my soul have not. I've simply forgotten to leave room for them in my busy, busy life. Everyone has his or her own vices, and I encourage you to re-discover and allow them back into your world. Make time for the things that feed your soul. These elements give you the power to create art.

3) It's OK to experiment.

One thing I am proud of is my ability to try, experience an utter failure, and have the courage to get up, wipe off the dirt, and try something else. I constantly experiment with new skills, projects, and ways of thinking to discover what is and isn't a right fit for my life. When things don't work, does it really mean I've failed? Oh, hell no.

It just means I have not found that one thing out there that is my true, unique, artistic calling. (Yes, I am still looking.)

I see too many people in this business think they already know everything and, in turn, try to force and control life's experiences. They think they are meant to be an actor, even if they are miserable and are meant to produce instead. If there is one thing that will block you from creating art—the art that speaks to *you*—it's ego. It's not easy admitting we don't know everything, and it's brutal not knowing what your purpose on this planet is, and whether or not we'll achieve success when we find it. And guess what? That search may take your entire life, and you may never be rich and famous, but that's okay. Art stems from experience, not success. If we keep searching for that path and doing what we love, someone, somewhere will surely be inspired.

4) Do the work.

If you haven't read Steven Pressfield's *The War of Art* you need to grab a copy and read it NOW. He uncovers our inner creative battles, and it's a must for any artist. Even when we are living in a state of calm and we learn to avoid the hustle, there is another element that stands in our way, blocking creativity from flowing: ourselves.

That's right, our own minds create so many distractions and unnecessary hurdles, from procrastination to a lack of confidence to the need to forever self heal. Pressfield walks us through the ways in which we resist actually *doing the work*. The art. The creations we fight so hard to find the time to do.

As an Aries, getting stuck in my head is all too familiar. I'm sure many of you can relate. You know, when you actually have the freedom to sit and create, and you end up spending 5 hours on Facebook instead. Or you just stare at a blank page, wanting every word to be brilliant. In fact, I put this article off for nearly a week past my deadline because I was afraid my words wouldn't be as inspirational as I hoped. Then I forced my butt into a chair (and did items one through three above), and vowed to sit here until it was done (and look, I am almost there!).

Pressfield's book encourages us to sit and "suffer" in those moments because it allows us to move past the resistance and into the depths of creativity. We can—and *will*—eventually train ourselves to get into this mode more often simply by forcing ourselves to do the work in front of us. After all, isn't that what we want to do? Create?

Lifting our spirits is not the responsibility of this city, of your agent, producer, or even life coach, though many people will provide incredible wisdom to you along the way. It's *our* responsibility to take care of our own soul, so that we create art and reflect that beam of inspiration back into the world. Trust me, once you are on that high and your energy is beaming, everyone will see that shining light and come running to it.

***

Showrunner, executive producer, host and brand expert **Kristen Nedopak** is the creator of the award-nominated *The Skyrim Parodies*, the first-ever award show for geeks, *The Geekie Awards*, and other innovative sci-fi/fantasy digital content. An advocate for independent entertainment, gaming, and art, Kristen is a public speaker for several organizations, such as *Women 2.0*—coaching women to become entrepreneurs and leaders in their industry. She a regular panelist for San Diego Comic-Con, WonderCon, DragonCon, GeekGirl Con and more.

PART TWO: Biz Basics - Set-iquette

The Call Sheet Cheat Sheet
By Erin Henriques

You've finally landed a role in a movie. You've received your first call sheet and excitedly spotted your name. Now…who the heck are all those other people listed on there, and what exactly do they do?

While I hope this post will be useful to readers in all aspects of the film industry, I'm specifically directing it to my fellow actors. We don't necessarily learn about the roles of a film crew in our college theater programs or ongoing scene study classes, but the truth is, production is a "team sport". Whether you're an actor, a set costumer, a 2nd AD, a 2nd 2nd AD, or a dolly grip, it's important to understand what all of the roles on a set are so you can be the best "team player" possible.

So, enough of this cheesy sports analogy. Here's a simple breakdown of some key people you might come across on a set. You could fill a book—many books, actually—with all of the complexities of each of these jobs, so think of this as a very basic breakdown: "A Call Sheet Breakdown for Dummi-er-Actors", if you will!

Production
Director: this is the captain, the leader, the department head of all of the department heads.

1st AD: the conduit between the director and everyone else on set. This is the person that calls "last looks", "picture is up", "rolling", etc.

2nd AD: reports to the 1st AD. Responsibilities include everything from creating call sheets, leading the cast through hair/make-up/wardrobe, and making sure everyone is on set when they need to be.

2nd 2nd AD/3rd AD: this is the position below the 2nd AD on large productions where more help is needed. A 3rd AD (or 2nd 2nd) will often help wrangle and place background.

Script Supervisor: watches for continuity and keeps a detailed log of filming. You will always find the script supervisor sitting next to the director and watching the monitor.

PA (Production Assistant): this brave soul does all the stuff that no one else has time to do or wants to do.

Camera

DP (Director of Photography): also known as the cinematographer. Works with the director to make artistic and technical decisions about the look of the film.

Camera Operator: physically operates the camera under the DP's direction.

1st AC (Assistant Camera): also known as the focus puller. The 1st AC measures and pulls focus for the camera operator. He/She also does the daily camera assembly and breakdown.

2nd AC (Assistant Camera): operates the clapboard, loads film, changes batteries and lenses, and manages logs and paperwork.

Sound

Sound Mixer: the Sound Department head. Oversees the recording of all sounds on set.

Boom Operator: uses a boom pole with a microphone on the end to record dialogue and action.

Sound Utility: assists the sound mixer and boom operator with multiple tasks, including testing equipment, setting up microphones, and pulling cable.

Grip

Grips are technicians who work with both the Camera Department and the Electrical Department to set up things like camera and lighting rigs, dolly tracks, cranes, etc. Remember *Fraggle Rock*? Well, grips are like Doozers.

Key Grip: head of the department.

Best Boy Grip: main assistant to the key grip.

Dolly Grip: specializes in setting up dolly tracks. Also, physically pushes the dolly with the camera (and camera operator) on it.

Lighting/Electrical

Gaffer: head of the Electrical/Lighting Department. Works with the DP to execute the lighting of a set.

Best Boy Electric: the main assistant to the gaffer.

Art Department

The Art Department runs deep. It's helmed by a **Production Designer** and an **Art Director** and is made up of various smaller divisions like the Set, Construction, and Paint Departments. You may not see the Production Designer, Set Decorator, and Construction Coordinator on set every day because there are times when they will be busy working on other sets for future shoot days on the movie. However, here are some of their representatives who cover the set daily:

On Set Dresser: places and organizes decorative items on a set. For example, he/she might hang pictures and arrange furniture for an indoor scene or place leaves and debris on the ground for an outdoor scene.

Standby Painter: watches the set and makes paint touch-ups and paint changes as requested by the director. He/she also handles any issues that may come up with wall hangings, signs, or finishes on different surfaces.

Props

The Props Department works within the Art Department in collaboration with the art director/production designer. This department supplies and arranges all objects handled by actors and portable property on a set.

Prop Master: the head of the Prop Department.

Assistant Prop Master: assists the prop master (Even the assistants get to be called masters! This department wins.)

SFX (Special Effects)

The SFX Department works with the Art Department. It is made up of an **SFX Supervisor** and **Coordinator** and supported by **SFX Techs**. These are the people that help create effects that physically happen and are filmed in real time. The SFX department handles things like explosions, squibs, and prosthetic dummies.

VFX (Visual Effects)

Like the SFX team, the VFX team also works with the Art Department and is led by a **VFX Supervisor**. The VFX Department is responsible for all effects that cannot be captured in a live action shot. This department handles things like matte paintings, miniatures, green screens, and CGI. While VFX completes their work in post, their jobs start on set. Department members are present during filming to do things like take pictures and set markers.

Wardrobe

On a large production, the Wardrobe Department might consist of a **Wardrobe Supervisor** and/or **Wardrobe Designer** (who may or may not be on set on a daily basis) and a team of set costumers.

The Wardrobe Department costumes the cast on a show, launders and maintains costumes, and does on-set dressing of the costumes (e.g., adding dirt or sweat stains as needed).

Make-up and Hair

Large films generally have both **Hair and Make-up Department heads**. They oversee design and lead their own teams of **hair stylists and make-up artists**. This department designs actors' looks, executes them on a daily basis, and then maintains them on set.

Both the Make-up/Hair Department and the Wardrobe Department are important for actors because we work very intimately with them. They can truly help bring our characters to life. Always remember to appreciate how these artists can help you with your craft!

Transportation

Transportation Coordinator: manages and oversees all of the transportation needs of a production, including the transportation of people and equipment.

Transportation Captain: works under the transportation coordinator and is responsible for transporting cast and crew to and from set.

Medic

Set medics stand by on set to help in the event of a medical emergency.

Catering

This lovely department provides meals!

Craft Service

This lovely department provides beverages and snacks *between* meals!

So there you have it. See you at the craft service table!

***

Erin Henriques is an actor and a writer. Originally from Los Angeles, she studied acting in Chicago (*DePaul University*) and London (*LAMDA*), worked as an assistant on a movie in Mexico (*Master and Commander*), and briefly lived in New York (it seemed like a serious actor thing to do). After amassing a lot of new life experiences and more than a lot of debt, she returned to LA where she's been working on film, television, and theater projects ever since. Some favorite credits include *Chozen* (FX), *Mandie and Earring*, shorts for Channel 101, and an improv game show pilot for CBS.

On Set Etiquette For the Beginner
By Katherine Di Marino

The following are some tips for when you are visiting, or working as a cast or a crew member on a set, when you're first beginning your career.

I'll start with probably the most important one. **Stay out of actors' eye-lines.** If you are there, you are a cause for distraction. The first time I visited a set I made this mistake and the actor pulled a Christian Bale and went ballistic! Try and stay behind the monitor if possible.

And then there is the subject near and dear to everyone's hearts: food! If you're visiting, **let the crew get through the catering line first—** particularly if it's a unionized crew. They have a set amount of time for their break and if you get in line before it's appropriate, you will get many glares burning through your flesh.

While we're talking about food, **don't stand all day grazing in front of the craft service table!** That food is for everybody and I've seen MANY people go to town because there are free treats sitting there in front of them. Particularly if you're a visitor—it looks really cheesy and gets noticed!

Once again if you are a visitor, **do not fawn over the actors or approach them without an introduction from your contact that has brought you to set and has given the okay to go ahead –** particularly if they are in the midst of an emotionally taxing scene. They will once again go mental on you depending on who they are and their temperament. It may not end up being the quaint meet and greet you were hoping for.

As with actors…**don't talk to the director.** He/she is usually focused on his next shot or scene and doesn't want people approaching for chitchat. So unless you've got earthshattering business to deal with, do not bother them!

If you need to sit, **do not do it in one of the directors' chairs**, especially if it has the director or producer or cast's name on it! Amazing how some people do this. Sit only if you are invited to.

Keep your eyes on your feet. Watch out for cables and equipment when walking. Sounds obvious but it can be like a minefield, and I've had a couple of trips myself. Sandbags are usually good enough to stop things from toppling over, but it can make for an embarrassing situation.

The minute "action" is called, keep your mouth shut and stand perfectly still. If you need to cough, stifle it, otherwise you won't be very popular. After "cut" is called you can do whatever you want, but for those few moments pretend you're a statue. I once worked on a studio shoot that was done in real time where the green camera operator was getting directions through a head set, and she started talking back to the producer in the booth in the middle of an interview…who of course could not hear her. Nobody was amused, and the host was apoplectic and couldn't hide it, although the cameras were still rolling!

Unless it's your job, do not touch the sets or props. This is a good way to get the art director, set dresser, and props man angry. Not only are sets and props not there for your touching, but there's often continuity (called a hot set), which you've just messed up! Now the continuity person can get mad at you too. (I once saw a writer take a sticky bun off the top of a plate and bite into it as it was being carried to the set for the next scene. People make mistakes—don't let it be you!)

Never stand in front of a light (or a silk that has a light shining through it). You will cast a shadow, which will make the DP go crazy on your backside as you've just re-lit the scene. A friend of mine learned this the hard way!

If you're on a low budget shoot, pitch in when necessary setting up and dismantling or moving stuff around because you're likely running with a very small crew. Don't be precious about it even if you're doing hair that day—everybody has to lend a hand. I've worked on a couple of projects where able-bodied men sat there and watched me move heavy stuff around without offering to lend a hand. Don't be that person!

If you're a member of the crew, save your flirting for the end of the work day. A director I know was almost blackballed for being more interested in the make-up girl than what was going on in front of the camera. A lot of tongues were wagging. I am aware of another director who invited his girlfriend to set for most of the shoot, and he will be remembered for his endless canoodling, not his film. So keep your head in the game. This is the stuff people remember about you and it makes a difference to whether you get invited back for future projects. Professionalism at all times is very important.

If you intend to bring someone to set, get the permission of the producer first (who will discuss it with the 1st AD and director). All visits should be authorized and will be noted on the call sheet so everyone is aware of who the stranger is in their midst and whether they belong there, and haven't just walked in off the street. You may have no idea what scenes are on deck for that day, and something sensitive like a sex scene could be on the agenda, which means a closed set. Or once again something particularly emotionally taxing for the actors and distractions will want to be kept to a minimum. It's up to the powers that be to decide what is an appropriate day.

If you're working on location, do not walk in and out of doors attached to the set when rolling. If you leave set, make sure to close the door tightly after you've departed, or the 1st AD will get pissy with you.

Also if you're on location, **be aware of what you're doing, even if you're not on set,** but are in an attached room or you're upstairs. I once worked in a decrepit old building and even one floor up you could hear footsteps that sounded like jackhammers and conversation down below. Be aware of your surroundings and be sensitive to your environment and the noise you may not be aware you are making.

While we're talking about noise **make sure to turn cell phones OFF before walking onto a set.** Anything that rings, beeps, buzzes, or plays annoying music should not be on. Someone forgot to do this once and in the middle of a pivotal scene the theme music for "Jaws" began to play. Once again no one was amused! Think of it like you're going to the movies and you're seriously going to tick some people off if you suddenly receive a call in the middle of the coming attractions. Check and double check!

If you're a smoker it's just like about every other place in the modern world. There is no smoking on set, or around the lunch area where people are eating. You will have to go outside and remove yourself a good distance. There is usually a designated smoking area accompanied by a butt bucket. Be kind and throw your butts into the bucket, not on the ground, because some poor AD in training will have to come around and clean up after you once the location is wrapped. Same goes for chewing gum, do not throw it on the ground…put it in the garbage. And if you can't find one, there is always one located next to the craft service table. If you can't imagine yourself scraping the mess off the floor, don't leave it for some other poor sod to deal with.

Pay attention to signage posted on the walls and doors. There may be things specific to that location. For example, if you're shooting in a high-end house, all food and drink will be prohibited to prevent damage to the Persian rugs. You may also be required to put cloth booties over your shoes just like movers do before stepping onto the set.

If you are an extra, never look at the camera! Never, never, never. I've seen this happen before where someone's eyes begin to wander when they're in the background of a scene. This stuff shows, and the director's not going to be thrilled to receive the dailies and see that juror number four kept staring into the lens—perhaps looking for their close-up? Do what you've been instructed to do—no more no less. I saw a still photo just a couple of days ago from a film I can't identify that stars Nicole Kidman. It must have been *Batman*, because she's staring up at the sky with a horrified look on her face. The novelty of the photo was the extra, who had decided he was going to become a featured part of the scene, is emoting full on with his hands thrust in the air over Nicole's shoulders—almost drowning her out. Background means you're in the background. If the director wants to feature you, you will be approached and asked to do something special, and your pay bumped accordingly because you're being featured in some way.

Always follow the production's instructions to the letter, even if you're just a day player. If you've been asked to come in a certain type of clothing do that and bring other options with you. If your hair is going to be styled make sure it's clean unless instructed otherwise! I've seen several actors turn up on set with hair so greasy you could fry an egg on it. Depending on the size and budget of the productions, running water may not be hooked up in the hair and make-up trailer. What can they do but sprinkle powder all over your head to make you look less like a derelict? It ain't sexy folks! Particularly when somebody else has to run hands through it! Don't assume you're going to get a wash and blow-dry unless you've been told so.

These are just a few tips and tricks of things to look out for if you are paying a set a visit, or starting your career and becoming more familiar with the dos and don'ts of on-set etiquette.

***

Beginning her career in 1994 as the Producer's Assistant on the TV series *Highlander*, **Katherine Di Marino** was eventually awarded an Associate Producer mentorship by the CMPA on the Showtime series *Dead Man's Gun*. She went on to gain a broad knowledge base throughout her work at *Peace Arch Entertainment* and *Omnifilm Entertainment* in the areas of development, production, and business affairs. During her career she has been involved on many projects including Francis Ford Coppola's sci-fi series *First Wave*, David Steinberg's comedy series *Big Sound*, the half-hour dramedy *Robson Arms*, five Lifetime Network movies, the animated series *Pirate TV*, along with nine documentaries. She also did two stints at Creative BC as an Analyst. She launched Max B Productions through which she is writing and producing her own projects with a focus on comedy and children's programming. She has done work for over 20 broadcasters and won numerous international awards.

Tips They Don't Teach Ya
By Paula Rhodes

This month (a rather hectic one for me, as it involves a move into our first little house after a year-long hunt) I have noticed a plethora of little gems of knowledge coming my way through the chaos. And despite an initial selfish thought to hoard them all, I'm going to share them with you. Use them well, my pretties, and may they bring us all much success!

For the most part these do tend to pertain to acting specifically, but some are transferable to various arts

1) Send thank you notes.

I know, it's a pain and seems outdated, but I personally have gotten more repeat auditions with casting directors specifically because of this than I can count. On a related note, Michael's craft stores have packs of eight cards for $1. Boom.

2) For film auditions—BE STILL.

Duh, right? But no, I mean really, *really* still. As in, don't move your head at all, be super grounded, and let it all come out through your eyes. You will exude a power and invite an intimacy that is key for film/TV and it will help you stand out. It does feel weird at first, but on screen it works. You may be directed to, or decide to move as one normally does once you book the job and are on set (depending on the material). But check out some of the most powerful performances in your favorite flicks—notice the stillness. Magic.

3) Be nice. Always.

Seriously, that jerk that cut you off on the 101 and you decided to flick off and honk at... kind of awkward when you have to read together for your audition that you were rushing to. Or worse yet, when you have to read FOR them. Always play the Grace Card.

4) Look beyond.

This is a fun little trick I wish I'd known earlier in my career. Directors, take note if your actors don't know it! When they're filming your coverage on a close up and you're staring lovingly or angrily or whatever into your co-star's eyes just inches from yours, it's most likely going to make you look rather cross-eyed. To avoid this, look "through and beyond" them at some point far in the distance. It takes some imagination, but when you're sitting in the screening looking at your 20-foot tall face sans crossed eyes, it will be worth it.

5) Your mic is on.

This one harkens back to point number three but covers a bit more ground. Once you're on set and your microphone has been clipped on (or even if there's just a boom being held off to the side—that sucker picks up LOTS), be aware that everything you do and say can be heard by someone. Everything. And you never know who has their headphones on—most likely at least the sound person, but perhaps a producer, director, or other key people. So ask to be shown how to flip your battery pack to "off" before bathroom runs, don't say things you wouldn't say to the whole set, and don't complain. Just don't.

6) Google it.

Use your time on set to learn. Don't know what a "gaffer" does? Wondering what they mean when they say they're shooting the next scene "M.O.S."? Wonder how many hours are left before lunch will be served according to SAG rules? While you certainly could ask these questions of the nearest crew member, you risk showing your greenness and potentially slowing down the set as they explain it to you. Use it as an opportunity to educate yourself and look it up.

7) Be a team player.

In this case, I mean like when the shot is on a close up of your co-star and you're either off camera talking to them or they're shooting over your shoulder with a just a bit of your body in frame ("dirty"), really be there for them. Give them at least close to the same performance you'd give in your close up so they can feed off of you and give their best take. Also, try not to step on or over their lines with yours in this situation so the editor has an easier time of cutting back to you. Now, this courtesy may not be reciprocated (which can be frustrating), and you may often find yourself acting out your emotional close up with a post it note on a wall for an eyeline and a P.A. deadpanning the other lines at you, but be a good example and be there to give whatever is most helpful to your fellow actors and director (which, sometimes, may also mean just heading to your trailer if they request it instead. Who knows, actors are weird).

8) Step forward.

This one seems a bit odd but works wonders. When auditioning, they often have you do a scene once, then give direction and have you do it again accordingly. While the CD or director is giving you notes, move just a little bit toward them (not too close, but enough to break through and become a human who is interacting with them). It shows you're interested in what they have to say and really listening. Take it in and then move back onto your mark to give take two. It also gives you control over when take two starts as they need to wait until you're back on your mark.

9) Technical Skillz.

Yep, with a "Z" cuz there's lots. There's a lot that goes into a good performance that directors and editors can help you achieve, but make sure they never have to make up for your snafus in these areas (or you're left hanging in situations where one of those positions is occupied by a less-than-magician). Make sure you and your co-stars have the same eyeline when watching that vampire/bounty hunter/hot guy in the distance. Know how to hit your mark when one is given to you (good peripheral vision!). Make sure continuity is on your radar and/or know how to utilize the script supervisor (i.e., if you pick up a donut with your right hand and take a bite immediately after you say the word "bumblebee", make sure you do that the same way/time in every take). Making it all look easy will come in time.

10) Be responsible.

This covers a lot. Aim to be a pinch early, not just right on time— never let the hold up on set be because of you. If you sweat buckets, remember to bring your super-powered Certain Dry and maybe a personal fan or blotting papers to set. If you can't always guarantee tears with your performance and your scene that day demands it, bring a tear stick in case they don't have one (they sell them at makeup stores like Namies and Cinema Secrets—they're small menthol blowers that will give you eye rain for sure). If you've got specific dietary needs and are shooting in say, Texas, plan ahead and make sure you won't starve even if the caterer forgets to accommodate you. Just be your own mother and make sure you're taken care of. Now, of course a great crew/set will have all this stuff for you, but juuuust in case there's a weak link in that team, cover your own bases.

Now get out there and do stellar work!

**

Paula Rhodes is an actor/producer with emphasis in the geektastic genres and a founding member of the 5'2" & Under Club. She counts among her best diary entries teaming up with Stephanie Thorpe to turn their life-long love of the comic *ElfQuest* into getting the film/TV rights to it, and getting to embody her fandoms as Wendy in *The New Adventures of Peter & Wendy*, Lady Door in the West Coast premiere of Neil Gaiman's *Neverwhere*, Zelda in Knights in Hyrule, and Skipper in *Barbie: Life in the Dreamhouse*.

10 Things Making Movies Taught Me
By America Young

I have been working on movie sets of all sizes and budgets for ten years. During that time, I have learned a few things that apply to production *and* real life. Art imitates life, and life imitates art and the making of art. Or something deep and philosophical like that. Either way I was thrilled to find similarities between filmmaking and the rest of the world. It made me feel less like a mystical, lawless carny, and more like a relatable member of civilized society. Which is nice sometimes. Usually though, I prefer to feel like an artistic vagabond.

Here are the things I learned.

1) The unfinishable qualities of water bottles.
Once someone drinks from a water bottle and puts it down, that water bottle will never get used again. And it doesn't matter if you buy the super tiny bottles or if you write names on them (that only works if you have a dedicated person for the job). The act of putting down the water bottle leads to an amnesia of where "your" bottle went, an absolute conviction that THIS bottle is not yours, or if it is yours, that someone with mouth herpes drank from it. Either way the meager damage to the environment is not worth the risk of cooties, so you get a new bottle and vow to not let that one out of your sight, until something distracts you. This happens anywhere people have disposable water bottles and are in a large group, and it drives me nuts. Anyone have any solutions to this?

2) Sometimes the people in charge are clueless.
Sex. Nepotism. Stupid luck. Bullshit artists. Unqualified, inexperienced, and undeserving people get in positions of power. It happens a lot in Hollywood but also in every career. And it sucks. Hopefully one day it will work in your favor. Until it does, just work

hard. Be a hard working, nice person to be around and you won't need nepotism.

3) It rarely has to do with you.

Even if the world revolves around you, which I have no doubt that it does, most likely someone in a bad mood (or good mood) is dealing with something not related to your world. I have watched actors between takes anxiously watch the heads behind the camera talk and shake their heads and exclaim emotionally. The actors watch and grow worried. They are certain that they did something wrong and will be fired for sure. They put themselves through their own personal hell only to discover that there is a lens flare that's frustrating the crew or a huge argument over what's for lunch. Whether it's your boss or the rude grocery clerk, chances are their mood has nothing to do with you. So don't let it affect your mood or day.

4) The law of first day scheduling.

The first day never starts on time or goes according to schedule. Don't panic. Whenever I get a callsheet for the first day of a shoot, I always smile fondly. Nine times out of ten we will not be anywhere near this schedule. No matter how big or small the budget. When you are starting a new project—whatever the career—things will not go according to schedule the first day (or the second day). But the third day—the third might be just right. (It won't.) There are too many variables that not even a mathematician PhD can predict and calculate. Mainly because most of those variables are human. We are a hopeful species and more likely than not are way too optimistic with our goals for our first day. Don't panic. Just take a deep breath and work through the incoming anxiety and self-disparaging thoughts. If you stay calm and clear-headed, you will find your precious schedule again (as long as it was a reasonable schedule) and all will be right with the world. Unless it's a one-day project, then over-schedule by double and you'll make half of your day, which is just right. (That is an example of production math, as vague as calculus but 30 times more useful.)

5) Do your job.

Do your job as well as you can, no matter what it is. You are part of a bigger machine. Show up on time. Be prepared. Do your job. Charlie Sheen being fired off *Two and a Half Men* has taught us that no one is irreplaceable. No matter what someone's job, it is important and necessary. Don't give the powers that be a reason to replace you by being lazy, entitled, or a dick.

6) Shit goes down.

Sometimes those can be the best moments. When everything you planned for months falls apart—people don't show, locations are not available, gear is MIA—you can be screwed or you can be brilliant. You can let it end you or you can take those months of planning and think of a genius solution that not only saves the day but makes it even better than you ever imagined.

The moments that always get the most laughs and emotional reactions in my movies are things we had to think of on the spot to work around an issue. My favorite moments on vacation are ones when everything goes wrong and we have to improvise. The moment people remember at a wedding is when someone trips and turns it into a bow. In *Raiders of the Lost Ark* there is a scene where an expert swordsman does an amazing flourish with swords, which was supposed to lead to a complex fight with Indy. But Harrison Ford was sick as a dog that day and was dreading the fight. So he asked, "Can I just shoot him?" This wasn't at all what was planned, but Ford was really sick and so they had to improvise. And it turned out to be a very memorable part of the movie.

When the box collapses leaving only a cloud of dust, you will be forced to think outside the box. And out of the box in that cloud of dust (which is a magnificent mixture of panic, adventure, necessity and creativity) is where honest genius lives.

7) Everyone has an opinion. Not everyone EARNED his or hers.

Know who to listen to. In the age of the internet, everyone feels entitled to tell you their opinion. When it comes to your work, not everyone knows what they are talking about. Most actually don't. Know who to listen to.

8) Set boundaries way before you reach them.

When you are on set with everyone watching and you are asked to do something that makes you uncomfortable, whether it is to fudge the union law, be nude, or cut some shots from your shot list, it's a lot harder to be objective. Make sure before you show up to work (or go car shopping or to teacher-parent conferences) that you know what your hard line boundaries are and stick to them. Know how nude you'll get, which shots you will not compromise on, how much verbal abuse you'll put up with from the parents, and what extras on the car you can live without. Be able to walk away if you are tested. Never need something more than your morals. Never.

9) The loudest person on set is not always the scariest or the most powerful.

This goes for parents and all work places. The more power you have, the less you have to use it. Yelling usually signifies feeling powerless. That's why children have temper tantrums. And that's why grown ups have temper tantrums, unless you are Michael Bay and you just like yelling.

10) Important people have to wipe their asses too.

Accidentally walking into a toilet stall (that wasn't locked) and being face-to-face with a childhood hero of mine mid-wipe brings me to my final point. Of course, look up to people. Of course, be inspired by people, but be careful of idolizing. It makes it seem like others are better than you, which can then intimidate you into paralysis rather than inspire you into action. No matter who they are, they spend time of each day sitting on a too-short porcelain bowl with their pants around their ankles making sure they are free of fecal matter. Next time you meet someone who intimidates or undermines you, try to guess which butt check they lean on when they are wiping. My hero leans left. Puts things in perspective doesn't it?

In conclusion, the fact that so many things that I assumed were only film production issues actually apply to many other situations just strengthens my theory that we are all human. We pursue different dreams and goals in life, but we still have things in common with each other no matter what.

So remember whether you are creating art, saving lives, or shaping young minds: label your frakking water bottles.

**

America Young - director and professional stunt woman. She has stunt coordinated/action directed feature films/shows and music videos for Katy Perry, Ashlee Simpson, Chris Cornell and Natasha Bedingfield, to name a few. She has directed two music videos, five shorts, three entire web series and episodes from two others. She is in post on a scripted comedy pilot, *Wrestling with Parenthood,* which she directed about professional wrestlers. She is an executive producer on the *Girls!Girls!Girls* project and founder of *The Chimaera Project* non-profit. America's first feature, a pop-culture comedy called *The Concessionaires Must Die!!* is soon to be released.

Being Proactive vs. Being A Problem
By Leah Cevoli

In this day and age, self-promotion, networking, and being proactive overall about your entertainment career is pivotal for success and longevity. It's a fine line, and there's a balance that I've talked about before when it comes to online promotion and contests. But what about out in the real world? How does one network or more importantly *connect* with folks in the industry at higher tiers, folks that have the power to hire you without seeming desperate or worse yet, like you have a few screws loose? The key is to be authentic, to be yourself, and to *relax*. Easier said than done, I understand, but let me share a recent story with you about an actor who may have talked himself out of an audition—for a lead role in a feature film that he had previously been guaranteed.

I'm a producer on a feature film that is gearing up for pre-production. The lead role is still open, and our focus is on scoring an A-List director. An actor, a working actor with a 10,000 IMDb score, has been hitting us hard for about nine months now for the lead role. He met our EP/writer at a networking event, and our EP guaranteed him an audition. He has alternated between multiple emails to the general movie account and Facebook messages to the film's fan page. Each time, we politely answer him that we're not casting yet.

Recently, he began a Twitter assault, tweeting how he was perfect for the film and how much value he would add (*ahem*). Our executive producer got wind of this and sent the following in an email, with all producers cc'd:

> "We haven't forgotten about you. But we are right in the middle of picking a director, and this is not the best of times, frankly, for you to be trumpeting your interest in XXXXX. I'm the Exec Producer on this film. No one gets

cast without my sign-off, and I was the one who noticed you first. I haven't forgotten you. But please back off; keep bugging my producer and I'm likely to have a memory lapse. Just relax. You're in a good position right now. You will get a chance to read. Don't f**k it up, okay?"

RELAX!!!! You will either get to audition or you won't, but if you consistently bother the producing team for nine months, after they have repeatedly told you they weren't casting yet, you are changing from being proactive to being a problem.

In a situation like this, where you are one hundred percent sure the team knows who you are, and the executive producer has already expressed interest, the best thing to do is to stay in their minds via a presence on their social media pages. And by that I mean clicking "like" on things like the production posts, re-tweeting and sharing, and participating in the conversation. Not only will that keep you fresh in their minds, but it also shows you care about the project, you're engaged, you're participating, and you're sharing with your own network. Popping up every couple of weeks with private messages asking when your audition is shows us that you're not interested in anything but your own gain.

Here's another example, but this time we're not talking about a desperate actor, but rather a "few screws loose" writer.

A few years back, I was attending a convention in support of a television show that I had been acting on. The show creators were in attendance and I was still very new to the show and their circle of friends. I felt honored to be their guest at the convention, and like a kid in the candy store, I was excited to hang out with them at their signing table and in the green room. Enter crazy lady.

A few weeks prior, a woman I had met years earlier at a nightclub contacted me to say she was no longer working in music, she had left her job at MTV and was looking to represent and manage actors. She remembered me, noticed that the TV show I was working on was appearing at the convention, and hoped we could meet up there. She invited me to drive to the convention with her, and thank heavens I declined and drove myself there.

From the moment I met up with her, along with her husband and daughter, all she wanted to do was talk about this script she wrote, and how she thought the creator of the show I'm on would love it, and could I help her get it to him. I explained that this was my first time at the convention, and I was really trying to walk around and enjoy it, it was loud, it was crowded, she was blocking traffic trying to show me her script and could we meet up for coffee some other time.

I managed to get away from her for a bit and spend time with the folks from the show. And then she showed up again, just as announcements were coming on that it was time to leave. At this point, I'd been invited to the green room to hang out for a bit before leaving, and this lady tried to follow us, inviting herself, and her husband and daughter too. Finally, when security realized she wasn't exactly with us, they escorted her and her family outside.

A little while later, I was sitting in the green room with one of the show creators when one of the crew came in and said,"Man, this crazy chick in the parking lot, followed [other show creator] all the way to his car and kept asking him to look at her script!"

I kid you not. My mouth dropped open, I looked at the friend I was sitting with (who knew this lady had been stalking me), and he just shook his head, telling me to just act like I had no idea what they were talking about. But I was mortified. I made sure to call my friend the next day to apologize.

So, what's the lesson here?

Don't be a persistent problem, but also be very wary that you're not hanging out or associating with problem folk or, in this case, those with a few screws loose.

At the end of the day, your reputation and your resume are all that you've got. You can get by with a shaky resume, but you can't get by with a shaky reputation. There's a familiar quote, "People won't always remember what you did, but they will remember how you made them feel."

Be smart about networking, be authentic, and realize that strong relationships are built over years. It takes time, so don't try to rush it.

***

Leah Cevoli is an actress, host, and producer of film, television, and web, including appearances on *My Name is Earl* and *Deadwood*. As a voice actor, she is most notably known for her work on Cartoon Network's *Robot Chicken*. A professional live event host, Leah has hosted thousands of rock n' roll concerts and fundraisers. She is also the founder of *All Shapes and Sizes Welcome*, a travelling group of women who speak at conventions nationwide. Leah offers practical one-on-one sit-downs to discuss your career roadmap via her *Coffee Chat Consultations* and has a reputation for crowdfunding success. She is also an experienced yogi, a beginner fire dancer, and a certified level two Reiki practitioner.

PART THREE: The Practical and The Tactical

Be a Lady, Not a Stereotype
By Allison Vanore

Every once in a while I get asked how it is working as a female in this business. What they are really wondering is, do I find myself passed over or treated badly by males in the film industry just because I'm a woman? That question always takes me off-guard. I don't ever really think to myself as I'm working, "He just said that to me because I'm a woman." It just isn't in the forefront of my mind. Some might say I'm naive, but I hope it's because I'm being myself and that I've earned respect among my peers as a good producer and not a reputation as a "female producer". I do know, of course, that female stereotypes and sexist behavior does exist. We are in an industry where the majority of those in working positions are male. But this industry has plenty of room for women of all skill sets and personalities.

Now I will admit to one thing that I consciously do, and that is to make sure my actions and responses don't reinforce the stereotypes that haunt women in business—the idea that women are crazy, emotional, and/or bitchy. Because I don't consider myself any of those things, I make an effort not to say or do something that reflects those characteristics. If someone asks me how things are going, I make sure not to respond with "I'm crazy right now!" or "I'm flipping out!" And I definitely try not to publicly vent about things being out of control or bad (especially not on social media, ladies!!). While it's okay to get flustered and overwhelmed (we all feel that way at some point—and men do too!), it's about making sure our image and reputation aren't clouded by those real but momentary states.

So think of it as personal PR. You don't want to be remembered by those negative adjectives, which will unfortunately perpetuate the stereotype and potentially hurt us in the long run. From the beginning, I vowed to create my own story and control my image. The story I choose to put out there is that I'm busy, organized, under control, and work hard to tackle anything that comes my way. And I think it's working.

***

Allison Vanore is an award-winning webseries and feature film producer with notable series such as *Anyone But Me, My Gimpy Life,* and *Producing Juliet.* Her feature film credits include romantic comedy *Hopelessly In June,* horror comedy *Love in the Time of Monsters* and upcoming dramas *Daddy, 42 Seconds of Happiness* and *Depth.* Allison is also the Course Director and Instructor of Producing Independent Film at the Los Angeles Film School in her spare time—of which there isn't much!

Finding Your Voice
By Katherine Di Marino

Whether you're a writer and want to show-run your own series, or you're a producer that needs to speak up when a broadcaster isn't quite catching the drift of what you're attempting to accomplish, or you're a director yelling action and cut, having to find a language and shorthand to speak with your cast and crew—or any role for that matter where you have a vision that requires the involvement of others to see it come to fruition—you need to be a strong communicator. All of these roles involve developing your own voice and making sure it's being heard. That involves speaking succinctly, passionately, truthfully, and in thoughtful considerate ways. Communicating is an art form that only improves with time. Plain and simple!

Throughout your career you will find yourself scratching your head at intervals, walking away from interactions wondering what the hell just happened. Your point, wishes, and desires seemed to have gotten lost somewhere along the way. This is a natural part of the growth process. Don't be scared of it. And never be too frightened to ask for a second kick at the can. If your needs aren't being met, or you're not being heard, or you think you sucked for a few moments, take a deep breath, shake it off, and go back in for another round. Asking for another meeting or another conversation or another take is perfectly allowable. It means you're asking for what you want and are not compromising, and most importantly you're being accountable to yourself and the other members of your team. It's important to make sure we are being heard properly and understood—and sometimes that rough territory just comes with the domain of having been born with breasts.

At the beginning of my career, meekness ruled the day. I was scared to voice my concerns, and to fight if necessary to get my point across. It was easier to back down and not be seen as being an uncompromising b-i-t-c-h—yes, that dreaded word. It took me years to figure out that there was a right way and a wrong way to communicate. And my way never involved raising my voice, insulting others, or making demands people weren't capable of meeting. That just wasn't who I was as a person, yet I still dreaded having to go toe to toe with someone while fighting for my ideals, beliefs, and vision. I got all fidgety and my eyes danced around the floor while I droned on about why I didn't agree with the source of my angst. Once I got some years under my belt, and owned the fact I had as much right to be in the room as the next guy, things became much easier. It took some time but it happened. The more you do, the more you prove yourself, and the more you begin to trust your own voice and ideas…. and therefore you're willing to fight for them.

My big first trial was on a documentary project, and one of the broadcasters was making wild requests that we could not possibly accommodate. Instead of getting into it on the telephone, I opted to write a letter instead, because that's where I'm at my best: when I can put my ideas down succinctly and efficiently on paper. It was the longest letter in history, but I did what I set out to do, which was to get them off our backs and let us do our jobs—delivering a compelling hour of television. And we accomplished that. That taught me another thing. If you are just starting out and haven't yet learned how to put your game face on, write an email instead. It buys you time, allows you to play around with what you want to say, and you get to make sure you're using efficient language that can be understood by a monkey. There's no room for confusion. I realize sometimes this isn't possible and there is an immediacy to what's happening and you've got to roll with it. But if you've got the luxury of a bit of time, step back and formulate what it is you want to say and why. Build your argument and back it up with facts.

You should always remind yourself you have a right to be in the room and you worked your way into that opportunity. You've earned the right to be respected and to be heard. Your ideas are no less valuable than anyone else's. Opinions differ—they're just opinions. Everyone's got one and so will you. Never be scared to throw your hat into the ring because your idea might turn out to be the best of the bunch. If not this time, then maybe next time. You may be sweating buckets at the notion of speaking up on your own behalf, but it's the only way you'll ever win the game. If you're standing on the sidelines watching things happen that you're not happy about, it's a lose-lose proposition. You are letting yourself down, and whether you believe it or not you're letting everyone else down too because you're not giving the best of yourself. You're not present in the proceedings.

Television and film are collaborative efforts. They are about playing as a member of the team. Whether you are leading that team or are just a member, you have a responsibility to show up every day and put in 100 percent. As a female member of this industry, I realize that it took me longer to come to grips with the fact that despite all my efforts, sometimes I would have people stepping all over my toes anyway. The key is once I became more confident within myself I was no longer fearful about pointing out that fact, and asking them to stop either consciously, or sometimes unconsciously, crushing my appendages. I had to realize that it all started with me. If I didn't speak up I was setting a bad precedent that would set the tone for the rest of the production I was working on.

Sometimes part of being a good communicator involves tough conversations—the ones you'd rather avoid. Just remember never to play the blame game. If you deal with things yourself, right away, soon enough you won't be a seething mess by the time you broach your concerns. Once things become personal they get ugly. And you don't want to be dealing with ugly conversations because they are hard to recover from. If you are stating your case ("here is what I'm feeling and why") there is no room for argument. You are just speaking facts without any finger pointing thrown in. Avoid making things personal—it's the kiss of death. Keep your conversations about the business at hand and what is best for your project. If you can manage to keep your emotions under wraps and speak clearly and matter of factly you've won the battle. You will find in life that there are people who may not hear you the first time, and you may have to state your case again—but that's okay. The lines of communication are still open and at least you are talking—sometimes ad nauseam—but at least you're making your voice heard.

Depending on your personality type, realize that becoming a good and efficient communicator is a skill that can be developed over time. We all don't start out that way. Realize you are in a new arena doing things you've never done before and having the types of conversations you've never had before. Who wants to tell the craft service person the food sucks? I sure didn't! How can you expect to get it right in the beginning? You can't. You'll probably cringe a few times but the process is working. You learn from making mistakes. Expect to put your foot in it a few times. I did and I survived it and moved on— with a bit more wisdom under my belt ready and prepared to face the next hurdle that came along. Use your voice and don't be scared of it and how you might be perceived. As long as you're not shrill and aren't making decrees like the Gestapo, trust me you'll be fine!

***

Beginning her career in 1994 as the Producer's Assistant on the TV series *Highlander*, **Katherine Di Marino** was eventually awarded an Associate Producer mentorship by the CMPA on the Showtime series *Dead Man's Gun*. She went on to gain a broad knowledge base throughout her work at *Peace Arch Entertainment* and *Omnifilm Entertainment* in the areas of development, production, and business affairs. During her career she has been involved on many projects including Francis Ford Coppola's sci-fi series *First Wave*, David Steinberg's comedy series *Big Sound*, the half hour dramedy *Robson Arms*, five Lifetime Network movies, the animated series *Pirate TV*, along with nine documentaries. She also did two stints at Creative BC as an Analyst. She launched Max B Productions through which she is writing and producing her own projects with a focus on comedy and children's programming. She has done work for over 20 broadcasters and won numerous international awards.

5 Easy Ways to Give Your Body Language a Power Boost
By Kim D'Eon

What does your body say about you before you open your mouth? And no, I don't mean how does your body look. I mean, what does it say?

In life, and especially in showbiz, it's critical you know how to harness the power of your body language. The way you hold your body, use gesture and touch while interacting with others is the first way to put your *best foot forward* ... yes, I love a pun.

I've made a career in TV interviewing people, observing them and gauging their moods as soon as I meet them...and also *projecting myself* in a certain confident way. So, I've learned a thing or two about the importance of body language—not just in showing others how I want to be treated, but also that the way I hold my body can influence the way *I feel!*

Take a TV interview scenario for example: I know that if I walk into a room to meet someone and they're sitting cross-legged and arms folded, it's probably not going to go well. Obviously. You know this too. Those people are closed-off, literally. But, if they are leaning back, hands by their sides—or better yet, if they actually STAND UP to greet me—I know things will go well. They've shown me their warmth and confidence with their open body language. This all happens in the blink of an eye. I know you've all experienced this on some level.

So, if you want to connect with people and project your best, most empowered self, this is for you! Even if you're not feeling particularly confident in a stressful moment or meeting, you can "fake it till you make it" with these simple steps.

1) Smile.

Like yawning and laughing, smiling is contagious. If you've got a really important interview, person to meet or speech to make, it can be easy to forget to smile. You might walk into a room with a super-serious, get-down-to-business look. Smiling will actually make you feel a little happier and it's the first disarming and confident thing you can project as soon as you walk into a room. It shows people you are warm, trustworthy, and confident. A simple smile will help kick-start that connection and make people open to what you have to say. Besides, you didn't spend all that money bleaching them for nothin'... so, show 'em those pearly whites!

2) Master a good handshake.

It seems really obvious, but I have shaken a lot of limp, floppy hands. You know the kind—just the tips of the fingers—yuck! How can you really connect with someone who instantly retreats upon first contact? Not to mention the fact that I'm making a quick judgment about your lack of self-esteem. Where's the power in that? Master a good, firm, friendly handshake. Don't overdo it. That's also weird. Find your happy handshake medium. (If you're worried about your clammy hands, don't "sweat" it. Your lifeless handshake will be much more noticeable than a great, sweaty one.)

3) Reach out and touch someone.

When I'm talking to people, I'll often just reach out and touch their arm. It just happens naturally. I don't plan it. But, if it doesn't happen naturally for you, it's a good idea to try to incorporate it when appropriate. A quick touch on the arm or back lets people feel that I'm connecting to them in that moment. And I really am! Touch is one of our most powerful communicators—especially in this touch-phobic society of ours. Physical connection (no matter how brief) really stands out. Harness it and you will connect to people faster than you imagined. (Interestingly, some people don't actually like to be touched. If you've been paying attention to their body language clues, this can be pretty apparent. Maybe don't touch them. That will just be awkward for both of you. Body language and common sense are a nice pairing.)

4) Eyes are the windows to the soul.
Have you ever talked to someone who doesn't look you in the eyes very often? It can be very disconcerting! We need more eye contact, people! It seems to be a disappearing form of communication in this world of hyper-tech stimulation. But without eye contact there is no sincerity and no trust.

5) Be BIG.
So, going back to the beginning, when I was talking about first impressions, I described the impact of an open body versus a closed one in an interview situation. It's something you might not have thought about before, but the bigger we look, the more confidence we portray and the more powerful we feel! Sociologists and psychologists have proved it!

Imagine a peacock or an ape beating his chest or a puffer fish blowing up to fend off predators. In the animal kingdom it is pretty obvious that when one wants to assert themselves, they get bigger. Turns out, the same is true for us.

On top of looking more confident, holding yourself in this way can actually make you feel more confident. Check out social psychologist Amy Cuddy's awesome *Ted Talk* on the subject of Power Positions. Through her research, she's determined that standing in open, dominant "power positions" for even two minutes leading up to a stressful meeting or interview can reduce your stress levels and increase your confidence.

Change from the OUTSIDE IN, girlfriend! Try it!

So, when you've got that important meeting, speech, or job interview, look 'em in the eye with a big smile and a great handshake, sit up tall, spread your arms, uncross your legs if you can and rock on with your bad self!

***

An award-winning Canadian TV personality, **Kim D'Eon** has reported for and hosted popular and critically acclaimed shows such as: *Entertainment Tonight Canada, Food Network Canada's Family Cook Off, CBC's Street Cents, Marketplace,* and *The Hour.* Kim is also an Ambassador of Change with *CARE Canada* where she advocates empowerment for women around the world. She now merges her journalistic foundation and media expertise with her passion for real food and whole health to inspire others to eat healthy, live life to the fullest and laugh a lot along the way.

Ladies, Lower Your Voice!
By America Young

There is a shocking lack of women in the "above the line" positions in Hollywood, such as directors, directors of photography and so on. Now, perhaps I am naïve, but I don't believe that it is a conspiracy. Yes, I am sure the old white boys' club exists. Sadly, it always will. And that club has given us some amazing films. However, it has been my direct experience that men have always welcomed me as a producer or director or stunt person. It has been my experience that men have supported and helped me, never undermined or derided me.

We woman are still lacking an equal voice in this industry. I think that is simply because people aren't used to **hearing** our voice.

I was on set directing a web series about larping ("Live Action Role Playing") called *Damsels and Dragons* a couple of years ago. I had a male DP, AD, and 1AC. We had a limited location so we were trying to figure out the best way to get coverage. The four of us stood around discussing options. I said "Hey guys, how about we flip her and the camera around and cheat her coverage with the same woods in the background? I think it'll match." They stopped talking, looked over at me quizzically and then promptly went back to talking about the issue. As if I hadn't said a thing.

My producer, who was a female, was standing nearby. I nudged her and said, "watch this," and said exactly the same thing the exact same way. This time, the guys didn't even look up. My producer started to get pissed! I held her back. I cleared my throat, dropped the pitch of my voice down a couple of octaves and repeated myself.

I said (in my booming-est voice) "**Hey guys, let's flip the actress and the camera around and cheat her coverage with the same**

woods in the background? It'll match." Their heads popped up. They looked at me, thought for a moment and said, "Yeah, yeah that'll totally work. Good idea," and immediately started setting up the shot—COMPLETELY oblivious to what I had done to my voice.

My normal speaking voice is pretty girlie. It's higher. I frequently speak with bringing my voice even higher at the end of my sentences, which makes it sound like I am not as confident as I feel. I have found by using this new speaking technique, it is easier for me to be heard by those who truly want to hear me. And when I don't, they either don't hear or are quicker to discount/dismiss what I am saying.

Simple but important.

So here's my theory.

Most men want us around. Most men value our ideas and contributions. Most men appreciate what we have to offer. BUT MOST MEN AREN'T USED TO HEARING OUR VOICE IN THOSE POSITIONS. They are conditioned to a lower timbre. They communicate on a certain frequency.

I'm not saying we should change to fit in, I am just saying, before we go screaming SEXIST, getting our feelings hurt and fighting a battle of the sexes that might not exist, perhaps, just perhaps, we should remember that as women become more and more involved in the industry, we are still moving in uncharted waters. Both genders need to be retrained. As we learn to project our confidence in our voice, men will learn to hear it, and then…the movie magic we will make together…

To recap, **if you are feeling unheard:**

1. Stay calm
2. Ground your voice from your diaphragm, or even better, from your ovaries rather than your throat.

3. Clear out unnecessary qualifying words such as "**I think** it could **possibly** work if we try it this way **maybe**?" Instead speak with confidence. "It could work if we try it this way."

4. Do not go up at the end of your sentences. It's a period not a question mark. It's a confident statement, not a request for approval.

If they are still ignoring your brilliance or disrespecting you, then they are dicks. Don't work with them anymore.

***

America Young is a director and professional stunt woman. She has stunt coordinated/action directed feature films/shows and music videos for Katy Perry, Ashlee Simpson, Chris Cornell and Natasha Bedingfield, to name a few. She has directed two music videos, five shorts, three entire web series and episodes from two others. She is in post on a scripted comedy pilot, *Wrestling with Parenthood*, which she directed about professional wrestlers. She is an executive producer on the *Girls!Girls!Girls* project and founder of *The Chimaera Project* non-profit. America's first feature, a pop-culture comedy called *The Concessionaires Must Die*!!, is soon to be released.

6 Tips to Better Productivity
By Briana Hansen

I am a productive person. And I'm proud to say that without any hesitation. I'm not saying what I produce is always good content. Some of it's good. Some of it's great. And the rest of it… well, it is what it is.

But the point is, I've made a habit out of productivity. And some of my friends and peers have started to notice. Many have started asking me what my "secret" is. There is no secret. I work at being productive. I'm proactive about it. I pride myself on it. I practice it.

So I began looking at some of my own habits that I use to help continuously create content, and here are a few of the tips and tricks I came up with that could help you do the same.

1) Tools.

Like any other habit, you need to give yourself every advantage to be successful. And that means investing in the right tools. I use Evernote, Google Calendar, and a physical personal calendar every day. You're going to have to do some personal trial and error before you know which tools will work best for you. But if you're going to get serious about your productivity, look into the tools that productive people use. You can simply peruse the "Productivity" section of your local App store. Don't expect yourself to get more productive without the right tools, just like you wouldn't expect yourself to get in better shape without actually going to the gym.

2) Write everything down.

Get a notebook and keep it with you at all times. If you don't want to physically write something down, make sure you have a device you can at least record the idea on before it's gone. This is vital.

I can't tell you the number of times that I've had an idea come to me in a flash—a concept, a title, a connection, anything—and I think, "I'll remember that," to only later remember that I had an idea I wanted to remember but nothing else. I hate that feeling. Not because my idea was the best thing that could have ever happened, but because that idea never got a chance to be good or bad. It died before it got a chance to really live. And there's nothing I hate more than wasted potential.

So write it down in a small notebook. Put it on a Post-It note. Talk to yourself in a voice memo. Do something before you lose that flash of inspiration. The more you remember from those moments, too, the more frequently they come around. So when you've got a problem you know needs some work, you can trust that the answer will come—and you'll be ready to write it down when it does.

3) Force yourself to focus.

In a world filled with distractions everywhere, this is one of the most difficult productivity habits. Just now, after I wrote that sentence, I wanted to go check my Facebook profile again (I changed my profile picture today, guys. It's kind of a big day for me). But I didn't. I forced myself to focus. I actively practice the habit of staying on task even when I don't want to. No, I take that back—ESPECIALLY when I don't want to. That's the most important time to push through.

If you only have one hour out of your busy schedule to focus on your Magnum Opus, don't let it slowly get carved down by mindlessly meandering meaningless articles or staring at social media (even if it is profile pic change-up day). Even if there's something else you really do need to do—like respond to emails—don't do it during your creative time. Otherwise, you'll slowly dwindle away at your precious time and you'll never get to what you actually wanted to do. Then you'll get frustrated and it'll be harder to sit down and tell yourself to write next time because you'll associate the feelings of frustration with writing. And it's all a vicious cycle until you grow old and bitterly sad because you never got the chance to actually create the wonderful things you were meant to create on this earth.

Maybe I'm being a little dramatic, but you get the point. When I get into my zone, I warn anyone who may need me in the next hour that "I'm going in". Then I put my phone on "Do Not Disturb" and throw it across the room. And I shut off my Wi-Fi and play classical music. And if I need to, I set a timer. Then I force myself to sit there and type something. Anything. Just put words on paper. Judgment can come later. You'll find after a certain amount of time, you'll forget about all the ways you tricked yourself into focusing and you'll just stay in the zone without realizing how much time has passed. And when that timer surprises you and you can see how much you accomplished in one small chunk of time, it'll feel fan-freakin-tastic.

That method allowed me to, in one month, write a 10-episode web series while simultaneously creating a draft of my first full novel, doing daily vlogs about the novel's progress, continuing to write regularly for *Ms. In The Biz* and my own blog, while doing stand up and sketch comedy regularly and still holding down a full-time day job.

4) Time manage.

If you know me, you know I'm a little anal-retentive about my schedule. But you also know I'm organized and reliable, and that I get a lot done. And all that comes from my ability to manage my time really well. If you can learn to focus, you can learn to respect when it's time to do certain tasks. If it's time to write, write. If it's time to respond to emails, do that. If it's time to chill and hang out with friends, do that.

I color code my schedule. I maintain a Google Calendar that has basically my ideal schedule for the week and a personal calendar that has not only my schedule, but also other creative tasks I want to make sure get done. I update both of them regularly. I've found a system that works for me. You'll have to do some trial and error to find what works for you. But once you do, you can simply trust that you've made time for everything you need to do.

I don't find being extremely structured in my schedule to be limiting at all. In fact, I find it liberating because it allows me to be more present in whatever task is at hand because I know I've made time for everything I need to do throughout the week.

5) Accountability.

I hold myself accountable for the goals I've set for myself. If I consistently have to add something to the To Do list, I take a long look at why it's not getting done. Which means constantly re-evaluating my priorities. If it's not getting done because I keep staring at Facebook and wondering why so and so wrote such and such on blah blah's wall, I need to practice my focus better. If it's because I've taken on too much and simply cannot get to it, that's a different evaluation.

I also have learned the value of collaboration. If I get the ball rolling on a project and am lucky enough to be able to collaborate with some of my incredibly talented friends, I know that they're depending on me to do my portion of the work. And because I care about them and know I've promised them something, I'm more likely to do it.

Even if you don't have a specific project you're working on but just a set of goals, find a like-minded individual. You two can keep each other's goals in check, remind each other of your progress, and continue to challenge and push each other to your greatest potential.

6) Study the best.

Like anything else, productivity requires practice. If you want to be productive, practice it and study it like you would anything else. One person I suggest is Michael Hyatt. He's got a fantastic blog and podcast where he gives helpful hints all the time. And he produces a lot of content so he not only talks the talk, but he walks the walk. And I'll bet you anything he, like me, probably walks a little faster than most folks because he's got things to do. As should you. So get to it!

***

Briana Hansen is a comedian, writer, actress, author, and overall enthusiastic human being. Born and raised in the Midwest, she trained at numerous theaters including *The Second City Chicago, iO, UCB*, and *The Groundlings*. She tours with various stand-up, sketch, solo and improv shows nationally. She currently lives in Los Angeles where she constantly creates and produces a range of different (usually comedic) projects.

PART FOUR: Don't Hate, Collaborate!

How to Make Your Life Better
By Alex Santori

To my lovelies in the entertainment industry: I know I don't have to tell you this but, my child, you have chosen a difficult path. And at times it can seem like a big scary world out there, filled with backstabbers, naysayers, and emotional vampires. But never fear, booboo, I bear good news! While we can't change others and how they behave, we can certainly make things a bit easier on ourselves. BUT HOW?? Well, I'll tell you. (Don't interrupt—it's impolite.) Do just like those wily Care Bears do when confronted by that dastardly Professor Coldheart and his minions: band together and create a force field of positivity around yourself. (OK, so that's not exactly what the Care Bears do, but I liked that imagery. Leave me alone.)

Whoa, whoa, whoa, Alex! What are you saying? It sounds like you're turning a perfectly self-serving article of "How I can make my life better" into one that is selfless and all about "helping" others. Well, listen here, Negative Nancy, yes and no. I am about to share a short list of super easy examples of how to positively contribute to other peoples' creative lives… and well, do you really need any other reason than that? You do? Seriously? Fine. Uhm…something, something…do unto others…positivity begets positivity…dopamine…etc. There.

1) What's the word, Bird?
Share your insight and experiences, whether they are good or bad. This includes CDs, editors, photographers, makeup artists…the list goes on. Let's spread the word about those that are great at their jobs and love doing what they do! Not only to make sure that they keep working but also to give guidance to those who are looking for awesome peeps to collaborate with. (And avoid those that… well, should be avoided.)

2) Shake that moneymaker!

This might seem silly, and possibly a little annoying at times, but consider contributing to the Kickstarters of talented artists and projects you believe in, even if it's just $1 or so. (Come on, I know you spent more than that at Starbucks today.) But, if you really can't help contribute in a financial capacity to that super neat project, just click that handy dandy "share button" and let the love shine on. Helping to make someone feel supported goes a long, long way.

3) Were your ears burning?

If you see a breakdown or a job description that you think your friend or colleague would be perfect for, let them know! Encourage them to go after it. Trust me, once you are famous and super rich, you'll want your friends right there with you.

4) It's a girl!

The experience of making your first movie has a lot of striking similarities to being a new parent. Treat it as if they actually DID just have a baby. (The stress, the constant second-guessing, the sleepless nights…) So, bake a casserole, drop it off, and don't take up any more time than that. Or offer up your services. (Specific services. Not just the general "let me know if there is anything I can do"… uhm, yes. EVERYTHING! It's overwhelming!) Offer something specific like, "I'm free during the day this week, so let me know if/when I can pick something up/drop something off for you." Or see if they need an extra PA for a day. You get the idea.

5) Magical happy unicorn thoughts.

Once a week (or more if you're feeling feisty), send a quick personal message to a creative person in your life (or any person! I don't discriminate against the less right-brain-inclined). And whether it's via Facebook, text, or carrier pigeon, let them know how they impact you/your creative life in a positive way. (I've gotten one or two of these sorts of unsolicited messages, and I can't even begin to tell you how AMAZING it feels. Those good vibes carried me quite a ways.)

This list is by no means comprehensive. There are many ways to share love and support to those around us. And don't forget, all of this mushy gushy lovey stuff goes two ways. If you need it, don't be afraid to ask for help! Give someone else the chance to feel like a superhero. Just remember to be genuine and effusive when it comes to saying "thank you"!

OK, my kids and kittens. Go forth, live long, and do good! XO

***

Alex Santori is delighted to be working with *Ms. In The Biz* in creating supportive, female driven content. When Alex was just a wee lass, she cut her teeth on the boards of the stage. Then she got her braces in voice/opera and subsequently wears white strips for film and television. When she's not writing or performing, she spends her weekends wrangling wild Spotted Lemurs on the mean streets of Los Angeles.

It's a Small Town...Always Be Kind
By Alexandra Boylan

The other day I found myself in a three-hour wait at the DMV. I had visited the DMV earlier in the week only to discover I had to take a test and didn't have the time to do it that particular day. So now in the DMV, on this random Tuesday afternoon, I stood in the back of a crowded room filled with aggravated people constantly checking the time. I happened to be standing next to three gentlemen who struck up a conversation with me. I won't lie, if I was to have met these men on the street at night, I probably would have walked in the opposite direction. But feeling pretty safe in the company of over a hundred people, I engaged in conversation with them. They encouraged me not to worry about my test and that I would do fine, as I sat there flipping through the manual, viciously trying to memorize a lifetime of driving in a couple of hours. We all chatted for a while and then, one by one, their numbers got called and they headed into the test room.

A few minutes later, one of the younger men came back to me, very excited that he had passed his test. I congratulated him and shared in his extreme excitement to pass the California driving test. Then his face grew serious and he said to me, "I'm really happy I passed this test because I was just released from prison twelve days ago after serving eighteen years of a life sentence for a murder I didn't commit." WOW! Well, you can only imagine my face after hearing this—complete shock. He shared that he was thirty-eight years old; he had spent most of his life in prison. Then he reached out his hand to mine and I shook it and he said, "Thank you for talking to me today and being so kind to me." He walked away from me, and my jaw was on the floor. I couldn't believe he had shared his story with me, and this experience really struck me to the heart. It was such a beautiful reminder of how important it is to always be kind to everyone you meet. You have no idea the day they might have had. Then my number was called, and I hustled up to the desk only to discover I did not have to take the driving test. This was not a random Tuesday afternoon. I believe I was meant to be there that day to meet this man.

What does this have to do with the film industry, you might ask?

My answer: EVERYTHING!

I feel this story rings true in the film industry because it is extremely important to be the kind of person that people enjoy working with. HUGE studios do not run Hollywood. Hollywood is run by people and the relationships they have with each other. You never know who you are going to meet and how they might come across your path in years to come. Always treat people with kindness and generosity—like the saying goes, "treat people as you would like to be treated." That's why you always see the same names popping up on films; these people enjoy working together and sometimes that might even beat out talent or money. I have worked in the film industry since I was seventeen years old and have always tried to keep this in mind: everyone I meet today could affect my tomorrow. Plus I really love working on films, so for the most part I feel complete joy when on a movie set. But I have watched others complain and bring down a crew, and I have always thought it was detrimental to their own experience and their future of working with those people again.

Many years ago, I struck up a friendship with an assistant director named Justin Jones while I was waiting on him at a restaurant. A week later, he called me and offered me a very small part on an *Asylum* film he was working on. The part only had two lines, but I jumped at the opportunity to get to play make believe. I only had one day on this film but lucky for me I met the director, Leigh Scott. About a month or so later, I got a call from Leigh offering me one of the lead roles in his new film. I was beyond thrilled and got to go on location for a couple of days where I met friends that are still dear to me to this day. On set I met the lovely Sarah Lieving and she said to me, "Did you know Leigh wrote the script with the actresses he wanted in mind?" I shook my head, thinking of course not, feeling extremely honored. Sarah said, "Leigh really liked you and wanted to work with you again." I was completely taken aback since I had only worked with him one day. While the conditions hadn't been the best, I never complained and fully enjoyed the experience, always with a cheerful attitude. People want to work with someone they like, no drama, no fuss. If you're going to be on location together for awhile, it is very important to have no divas on set. This goes for men and woman! No divas allowed!

This story resonated so deeply with me that I still think of it today. I am thankful for every opportunity that arrives and am always looking for new friends to collect along the way. Everyone is building their team and I know I am always looking for easy-going people to work with. On the set of our feature film *Home Sweet Home* we all lived together in a house and it was important for us to have a group of people that were a pleasure to be around. The movie would never have turned out as well as it did if we had not had so much fun working together. Our camaraderie translated into the film.

While John (the director/my husband) and I were embarking on the adventure of selling that feature film, we met with our potential future sales reps. Our decision to not sign any paperwork before meeting them in person was because we wanted to see what kind of guys they were. It was very important to us to make sure we liked them before we put anything in writing. When we met Ryan and Jonny from *Instrum International*, we immediately knew these guys were going to be our friends.

After they sold our movie at *AFM* to *Image Entertainment*, I was warned repeatedly from other filmmakers to watch out for sales reps and distribution companies. Horror stories started flooding in from different people about how their sales reps had screwed them over. John and I didn't worry. We just decided to trust in them and thus far had been extremely happy with our relationship. We took them out for drinks as a thank you. And anytime we had questions, they returned our emails promptly. They have proved their loyalty to us and have gone above and beyond on our behalf. The other day one of my sales reps and I got together for breakfast to discuss our next project. Halfway through our chat, I stopped and literally took his hand in mine (yep, I'm really sentimental) and said, "Can I just tell you how thankful we are to work with you? I have heard so many horrible stories from different filmmakers that got really messed over by their sales reps, and I feel the complete opposite, I love working with you and feel blessed every day by our relationship."

Ryan's response was, "We feel the same way about you guys. Do you know how many sales reps complain about the producers of their movies being difficult to work with? When we sign a movie, we really sign people. That's why we only pick a select few and most important that we like the people."

I could go on and on with so many more stories of how kindness spreads like wildfire and brings beautiful outcomes to those involved.

I have witnessed some really horrific treatment of people on film sets. I have yet to understand why or how these people think this behavior will benefit their film or their future. In all aspects of life, how we treat people will always come back around. Whether you're the boss or the person who gets the coffee, kindness will get you where money never can, and a rotten attitude will halt you in your tracks.

This business is completely built upon relationships, so protect them with all your might!

It's a small town ... always be kind!

***

Alexandra Boylan was born and raised in Georgetown, Massachusetts, where she first began her exploration into acting, which led her to relocate to Los Angeles. After working in the industry, she soon realized her true calling as a producer. She co-founded *MirrorTree Productions* which has produced two feature films, *Home Sweet Home* and *Catching Faith*. Alexandra is also the Co-Creator of *Your Perfect Adventure* which just released the first of its kind live action, movie, app game, *Your Pizza Adventure*, which brings a new

71

platform of entertainment to the world, melding video games and movies into one. She is an active member of Women in Film in Los Angeles and hopes to continue to create strong female-driven content for audiences everywhere.

US vs. THEM: Be an Actor They Want to Work With
By Hayley Derryberry

When I talked to some of my actor friends about working on the project *Red, White, and Bluey*, I got questions like: are they flying you to Australia? Are they putting you in a hotel? Are they paying you overtime or travel days? These kinds of questions get asked all the time, but for the first time it sounded strange to me because I didn't think of the production I was working for as "them". The director was a good friend of mine, so it felt like I was working on one of my own projects, and I realized that as actors we tend to create a distinction between the production and ourselves that shouldn't be there. As an actor, if the project does well, so do you. So why is it that as soon as we're hired to work on a movie, TV show or web series, we think of all the things "they" need to do for us? You should work with the production toward a mutual success, and that will make you someone "they" want to work with in the future.

I am guilty of this myself. Early in my career I played a villainess on an awesome zombie Nazi movie, and I made a total ass of myself. This was only my first or second major role in a feature film, and I actually got paid. I was really happy to work on the project and I loved the character I was playing, but on the last day of shooting, I got into a heated argument with the director/producer. I acted like a petulant child, and the result is that I lost all contact with the filmmakers, and while they left my part in the movie, they haven't given me any credit for it. Now that I've been a producer myself, I don't blame them for that outcome one bit. I totally deserved it, but thankfully I have learned from that mistake, and I am not that kind of actor anymore.

I got my comeuppance when my husband and I produced our first feature film, *Rabid Love*. We thought that all of the actors we hired were passionate about the project and happy to be working on it. We explained at length that it would be shooting very "guerrilla style" and they all said repeatedly how low maintenance they were and how they weren't "those kinds of actors". For most of them it was the truth, and I will gladly work with those folks again anytime in the future, but for a select few, it was not the case. Now I don't think they lied to us, I just think that when they stepped on set some other mentality kicked in where suddenly we weren't mutual collaborators anymore, we were their employers, and then it was "Us vs. Them." Suddenly their "low maintenance" turned into "Why isn't there a gluten free option for lunch today?" and "I'm not wearing those pants because they make my ass look big." On the flip side, one of our actors was so awesome—he helped us build props and sets. Another froze her booty off drenched in blood without complaint. Those are the little things that make producers say, "Bring back that actor we worked with on the last project".

Here are some things you can do to help make yourself an actor "they" want to work with:

1) Be passionate.

The filmmaker knows that no one is ever going to be invested in her movie as much as she is, but the one group of people who really should be is the actors. The actors have the most to gain from the success of a film because their names and faces are attached to it. So when you get hired to work on a project, be passionate about it. Do things like making it a point to meet the people you'll be working closely with and offer to do things like bring your own clothes as wardrobe options. I just worked on a movie where the lead actress brought a ton of her own clothes and it really helped out the wardrobe department, allowing them to stretch their budget further than they would have. Then, show up to work early every day with every line memorized and a continued passion to make this the best movie you've ever made. That kind of gung ho-ness will make you an absolute pleasure to work with.

2) Be low maintenance.

I just went to a screening of the show *Lone Target* on Discovery Channel, and one thing the producers raved about was how great working with the host of the show Joel Lambert was. He is a former Navy Seal, and the producers talked about how willing he was to work in insane conditions without complaint and how that made him someone they wanted to work with even more. Now you may or may not be a Navy Seal and therefore able to put up with rigorous physical abuse, I don't know, but I think my guess is pretty solid that you're also not a royal princess; so don't get on set and act like everyone needs to bow to your every whim. It sounds ridiculous, but you might be surprised at just how many actors show up for work and suddenly forget how to tie their own shoelaces. Don't be "that kind of actor". If you're working on a low budget project and you have a special diet, bring your own snacks to set. And even though people are asking you all day what they can get for you, you don't have to request things. If you have the time, make your own trip to crafty to get coffee. You could even do one better and bring some coffee to one of the crew who is outrageously busy.

The tone on set is almost always set by the lead actors, and you can tell a big difference when you walk onto the set of a show with cool, laid-back actors and one with uptight, high maintenance ones. The former has a happy efficient crew, while the latter feels like stepping into a funeral home or worse, a war zone. So be happy that you're working and share that happiness with those around you.

3) Promote yourself.

The last one is something you do even when you're not working on a project. I added this because when I asked an actress friend of mine how her "online presence" was, I was surprised to hear her say that it was nearly non-existent.

As actors there are so many factors outside of our control that decide whether or not we get hired, so it is really important to take charge of the ones that we do control. You've got your headshots, you're taking your classes, all there is to do now is wait for the phone to ring saying you've got an audition, right? Wrong. Don't wait for somebody else to build your career, do it yourself. Get online and connect with fans or potential fans, anyway. You need to have an online "you" that is your professional self and separate from your personal self. I think Twitter is a really great platform for this. Natasha Younge has some amazing blogs on *Ms. In The Biz* with great advice about using Twitter as a promotional tool, so check those out. Promoting yourself online makes you someone "they" want to work with because it shows producers that, if hired, they will get additional promotion of their project through you. Success of every movie, TV show, and webseries is contingent upon word of mouth, so if you are always getting the word out about what you're working on and you have an audience who is listening and responding, then you are a value to any production.

Now slap these three qualities on top of being a talented actor and there's no way you won't find success in this town.

***

Hayley Derryberry grew up in Tennessee and has been acting since the age of six. She and her husband Paul moved to LA in 2011 and produce together with their company *Rogue Taurus*. Hayley went to Sundance 2014 with the critically acclaimed film *Frank*, and has been booking small roles on television. She stays close to her indie roots, playing diverse characters in everything from comedy to horror. In fact, in *Living Dead Magazine,* Hayley was named one of the top five new Scream Queens and Rising Talent of 2014. Aside from acting and producing, Hayley is also a full time blogger/vlogger for *Alpine Village* in Torrance, California. With wholesome Midwestern looks, fierce talent, and a funny name, Hayley Derryberry is making her mark in Hollywood.

A Common Creative Goal
By Cat Doughty

It's 2008, the day before we start shooting on the first indie feature I've ever worked on. I'm standing outside a two-bedroom crew house awaiting the arrival of the last nine or ten people who will call it "home" for the next six weeks. Yes. Nine or ten people, two bedrooms. (What can I say, it was indie and we were on a budget.) I'm a lapsed theatre major, so I really missed the inspired tangle of artistic people coming together to create something. I was excited…and terrified.

When we, the three-person pre-production team, booked the house, I remember thinking that the experience I was about to have was either going to be absolutely amazing or truly horrific. In addition to the obvious "real world" scenarios playing out in my head (close quarters, a handful of strangers, and long/stressful days coupled with little sleep has got to be the prize winning recipe for drama), there was also the fact that we were embarking on a creative venture that would soon become public. All the hard work, the writing, the planning, the long hours we'd put in behind closed doors, it was about to become a real thing—an actual physical thing out in the world. You don't get to put a caveat next to your name in the credits that explains why you fell short. This movie would have to stand on its own. If we failed, we failed publicly. I hoped we wouldn't fail.

Without going into a million details, the entire shoot was something of a beautiful disaster. Most days, there weren't more than a dozen people on set, including actors. Each of us had more jobs than any one person has any business having, jobs that, on any normal movie set, would have been done by entire departments with experienced heads and crews of their own. There was drama and disaster, pressure and bad plumbing, laughably bad luck, but there I was, 5am, among the first to arrive, often last to leave, and even on the worst days, I can honestly say I woke up every morning excited to go back and do it again. I don't think that was the case for everyone, but in the end we all stuck it out and worked through the problems. The movie isn't great. It's really not even that good, but I wouldn't say we failed. I'm proud we finished it and I wouldn't trade a second of the experience. I might not have come away with an amazing movie, but in making it, I became a better filmmaker and I met talented, passionate people I'll work with for the rest of my life.

In fact, on every project I've done since, even the smallest, silliest things, I've come away having met people with drive, talent and a good attitude—people I know I want to work with again. With every independent film I get to be a part of, I'm building a community of people around me who are hungry. They want to create, they want to collaborate and I get that wonderful high that comes with working toward a common creative goal. Incredible things happen when you surround yourself with talented people that want what you want. Together we are better than we are alone.

Five years later, very few people have seen my first feature film. It doesn't get me jobs or press, it hasn't been a "success" in the traditional meaning of the word, but you know what? Of that first crew, four of us work together regularly to produce new material. The others are more far flung, but when we see them, it's a fond reunion and we've helped on each other's personal projects. Those relationships are priceless. At the start, I was afraid to fail. Now I know "failing" is just part of the process, and the truth is that no experience is a wasted one. So I guess there's no such thing as failure unless you just don't do anything at all. And what fun is that?

***

Cat Doughty has a BFA in Art and Technical Theatre from *Whitworth University*. After moving to New Mexico in 2007, Cat joined a group of passionate independent filmmakers called *Black Shepherd Productions* and co-wrote and produced a dark comedic webseries called *Flock*.

She has recently relocated to Los Angeles to study television writing at UCLA and continues to work on screenplays for future indie projects.

PART FIVE: Conquering "The Biz"

The Worst Relationship I Have Ever Had and Continue to Have
By America Young

It's a first meeting/date. Most likely a blind date set up between someone who knows you both. You are super nervous. You've heard great things about this person and know it could lead to amazing things. If you are smart, you do a little cyber stalking to be studied up on them, which, if they are awesome, only makes you more nervous.

When you are dating someone you really want to impress and who holds the keys to your future happiness in their hands and they tell you that you are amazing, beautiful and everything they are looking for, it is the best feeling ever. And then they don't call. They say they will but they don't. You play it cool. You "check in" with them, and they respond with more flattery and assurances. You get giddy again and then you wait. And wait.

Sometimes, there is a second date. And sometimes it leads to a beautiful future together making sweet, sweet magic. However, the odds are not in your favor. They are not in anyone's favor. I mean, this is movie making we are talking about, and the chances of having a happily ever after in this relationship are smaller than finding Prince Charming on a white horse. I mean that, literally. It's easier to find a Prince named Charming that rides a white horse than have a secure future in the movie industry.

"So you're telling me there's a chance. YEEEEEEAAAAAH!"

And there is STILL a chance—so we soldier on. We keep taking those meetings with investors, casting directors, production companies, studios and other people that have the power to make our dreams or break our hearts.

"Welcome to Hollywood. What's your Dream?"

Last year I had met an investor for my feature. He liked the script. He liked my director's reel, what I had to say about the movie, and the out of the box way we were making the movie. He let us know a couple weeks later that he was in. We were ECSTATIC! Then radio silence. We checked in. He was still in, just needed the contract with us. We said, "Great! Send it over." Time passed, we checked in again. He sent it over to us telling us we can make changes if we need. We make a few minor changes and send it back. Radio silence for another month. We check in. He's on it and will get back to us. Another month...and so this continues. Every time we talk, he says just the right thing. He is smart, gets it and gets us. And then he's gone again.

And after six months of this, it hits me: I wouldn't put up with a man I was dating treating me this way. Why on earth was I doing it now? Yes, I wanted to work with this charming, smart man with money and make "movie babies" with him. Yes, I loved everything he had to say and suggest. Yes, his company and knowledge would be amazing for us. Except, it wasn't amazing until it actually happened. It was the promise of my Prince Charming but no concrete action of him and definitely no sign of a white horse. I had no idea if he really didn't like the project but didn't want to hurt our feelings, or if he really didn't have the money but was too embarrassed to say so, or *what* was really going on. But we needed an answer. So I drew a very pleasant line in the sand and never heard from him again. I wish I had done that sooner and saved us months of limbo.

Limbo. So much worse than "no". I used to think NO was the worst thing that could happen. But now I see NO just means "next option". The dream isn't dead; it just needs a different approach. People always say that you need to be able to take rejection. You don't. I mean, you do, but that's not the hard part. You need to be able to take constantly-holding-your-breath-with-hopeful-anticipation-of-your-dreams-actually-possibly-coming-true-maybe. Limbo. SO much more exhausting than rejection.

I really do think someone could limbo you to death. (Limbo: the act of keeping you hopefully waiting, not the act of making you backbend under a pole to musical accompaniment. Although, I can see that being rather life threatening as well if you don't stretch properly.)

So now I approach this charming, sweet-talking, dream-making person that we call The Industry as I would anyone I was dating or friends with. Actions speak louder than words. If they really mean it, they will act on it. If they really want it, they will "put a ring on it." (Thank you Beyoncé.) I know that what I have to offer is valuable and if they can't see that (yet), no hard feelings. I move on to one with the foresight who does. And just like most people without vision, they will see you in a happy relationship and THEN realize what they missed.

In the meantime, do what you can to see your self-worth, empower yourself and stay out of limbo.

Death by Limbo is an awful way to go.

***

America Young is a director and professional stunt woman. She has stunt coordinated/action directed feature films/shows and music videos for Katy Perry, Ashlee Simpson, Chris Cornell and Natasha Bedingfield, to name a few. She has directed two music videos, five shorts, three entire web series and episodes from two others. She is in post on a scripted comedy pilot, *Wrestling with Parenthood*, that she directed about professional wrestlers. She is an executive producer on the *Girls!Girls!Girls* project and founder of *The Chimaera Project* non-profit. America's first feature, a pop-culture comedy called *The Concessionaires Must Die*!!, is soon to be released.

How Actors Can Build Their Personal Armor To Survive "The Biz"
By Taryn O'Neill

INT. TARYN'S CAR — 3:34 pm

Taryn stuffs her face with a protein bar as she speeds up La Cienega. iPhone ring cuts through music. She recognizes the number and hits the Bluetooth button.

                    TARYN

    Hey. What's up.

                    AGENT'S ASST.

    Hey Taryn, it's [redacted Agent]'s assistant. So they need to
    change your callback time today.

                    TARYN

    Seriously? To when?

                    AGENT'S ASST.

    From 8pm to 6:45.

                    TARYN

    I had to pull out of that panel to make this callback... and
    now they're changing with 3 hours notice??

SILENCE. Taryn realizes it's a redundant question. She sighs, glancing over to a red "mom" shirt on the passenger's seat.

TARYN

Fine. I'm on my way to an appointment but good thing I brought my wardrobe with me as I won't have time to go home—

AGENT'S ASST.

Great, thanks.

CLICK. Taryn takes a bite of her protein bar and keeps driving...DISSOLVE TO:

INT. TARYN'S CAR – 6:13pm

Taryn moves at a snail's pace along Beverly Boulevard. She touches up her mascara as she now dons her audition shirt and camera-ready hair. IPHONE RINGS.

Eyes narrow — answering

TARYN

What's up?

AGENT'S ASST.

They need to change your time again.

Beat.

TARYN

Do they think I'm a dancing monkey?

Awkward silence. (Taryn is rarely snarky on the phone.) But then the assistant snorts.

AGENT'S ASST.

Yeah, they probably do.

TARYN

So what time do they want me to be there?

AGENT'S ASST.

6:15.

Taryn looks at the clock.

TARYN

So they think I'm a MAGICIAN. It's 6:15 NOW.

AGENT'S ASSISTANT

It's... 6:15. Yup, it is.

TARYN

Well I'm in awful traffic so you just tell them that I will get there when I get there.

Click. This time Taryn hangs up.

INT. CASTING OFFICE – 6:25pm

Taryn walks into the casting office. For lack of page space, I'll condense:

She's told that the audition is <u>different</u> than what she had done at the first call—and she is <u>next</u> to go in—and here is the girl who is to play her "daughter"—*Door opens...*

Off Taryn's face as we FADE TO BLACK.

True story.

Guess what? The callback went awesome. I was funny, engaging, and had a director who seemed really interested to work with me. He and

88

the clients just seemed to like everything I was doing. None of my earlier frustrations had entered the room with me.

I didn't book it.

<u>This is my life as an actor and it made me want to write this post</u>.

The media portrays acting as *glamorous*: Movie and TV stars, YouTube celebs... all living "the life": money, fans, excitement, glamour. Even some of us non-celebs active on social media publicize the "fun stuff"—photo shoots, meetups, conventions, a pic from our trailer from the gig we booked. But the reality of an acting career is different.

At the beginning, when you are waiting tables or slaving away at your "survival job", the industry doesn't give you respect. They hope that you fail so there is one less aspiring artist in town. You race around town to every audition you can grab, your bank account is drained from classes and headshots, and your parents are just wondering what they did wrong.

And even when you start working, you are still "hoofing it" like my experience recounts: material changing on a dime, last minute call times halfway across town, your personal commitments at the industry's mercy. And there are the ups and downs with your emotions—as your hopes and dreams (and livelihood) rest on these jobs that you are up for. You go through more rejection in a month than most people do in a lifetime. And then, when you actually book the job (yay!) and work on set—there is a whole other set of challenges that can befall you, especially being the new face on set.

So if the world of acting is a three-ring circus, how do you keep a level head? How do you not lose your mind... and your soul on your way to a steady gig? <u>Build your own personal badass set of armor to navigate the battleground.</u> These are some of mine:

1) Have a badass mantra.

You are a professional artist. You are not an aspiring actor or a starving actor. Whether at an audition or on set, you must think of yourself as a fierce, trained actor who is there to solve a problem with your skill—bring to life a character that currently only exists on the page or the storyboard to sell a narrative and/or a product. Not everyone can do this. Create your own mantra that inspires you and fills you with purpose.

2) Have an inspiring book with you at auditions.

(i.e., not TWILIGHT.) If there is a long wait at auditions, or if fellow actors are doing the 'what auditions have you been on?' chatter, read material that inspires you and reminds you of why you are an artist and storyteller. This also helps when commercials and co-star auditions or work tip into the demeaning realm—because you are playing certain stereotypes, like Bored Waitress or Bimbo Beer Babe, and thus you are often treated as such. But you are not that stereotype. Having a book that engages your brain and soul is a good personal reminder.

3) Know who the frak you are meeting and working with!

Contextual information (I've preached this before): Hollywood is a business. You would not go into an interview without doing some research on the person you are meeting with.

1. Auditions: if you are at a TV/film audition and have not met the CD before, research them. They may not always want to chat, but research allows you to not only find out the shows they cast, but their social media presence or their other talents. CDs don't get the respect they deserve from the industry (and actors being sycophants does not equate respect)—so value what they do and engage with them as human beings, not gate- keepers to an audition with the director.

2. On set: research the call sheet before you get there. Know the names of the key crew and creative members—see what the director and DP have done before—commercial directors shoot movies as well. You never know when being familiar or even a fan of the director's other work can allow you to strike up a conversation, ultimately giving you the

opportunity to create a more dynamic relationship with him/her, and even discuss the other projects you are working on—which makes *you* fascinating.

4) Be fascinating.

People gravitate towards people who are passionate about things in their life other than acting. As most of you reading this are "multi-hyphenates", don't be afraid to share your other focuses if the opportunity arises. And indulge your passion for non-related topics—you never know what may spring up because of it.

5) Don't go to an audition with the sole purpose of booking it.

Yes, that's what we want to happen but it's an outcome that is beyond your control. Seriously. No matter how great you were. Pick one goal that you can work towards in the audition that you can actually have a shot at controlling. Such as, "this audition I am going to work on my 'wise mom character' and own what that means to me – even if I don't have kids." Or, "this audition I am going to register everyone in the room and not let the camera guy rush me." That way, when it's over, you will feel accomplished—not focused on the outcome—and you will probably give a better audition.

6) Follow up—with yourself.

You are your own walking and talking business. Take yourself out for coffee or fro-yo and be analytical about the audition or shoot you just had—especially if it didn't turn out well. But don't beat yourself up—try to find the constructive criticism and learn from it. Then implement it the next time around. (See #5)

7) Visualize. Visualize.

There is so much chaos in the film business that auditions and film sets can be tumultuous places. It can throw you off your game, especially if you are not regularly working or auditioning (auditioning is a muscle!). People who work all the time have a certain comfort level both in the audition room and on set. Those who are desperate, who are newbies, or just rusty, stick out like a sore thumb. Anytime I have a big audition, I visualize the entire audition, from getting into the car to walking out of the casting building. I familiarize myself with every emotion that could wreck havoc with my performance. I experience it—the discomfort, the nerves—so I don't have to in the room. Even if you don't work all the time, it will help you feel like you do.

8) Have faith that your talent and hard work will pay off.

This might sound trite but you have to have a sense of spirituality to survive as an artist. There is no linear equation to success, there is often no rhyme or reason why you do or don't book something. But I believe that if you take action, and pour your heart and soul into your work, it will pay off in the long run. Just sometimes not how or when you imagined. That's all I can say. But I can almost promise it.

9) All these things will start happening naturally if you control your own career by creating your own characters and content.

If you wear the hats and create the stories that you want to tell, the acting hat won't feel so heavy, so precious. You will see the purpose for your character and serve the story—and it will no longer be just about being good. And in doing so, you will surround yourself with collaborative and supportive people.

10) Give yourself a break.

Sometimes it is ok to cry, scream or laugh at yourself. Sometimes it's ok to be snarky to your agent's assistant because what they are relaying is ridiculous or frustrating. Crawl into bed, down a bottle of wine or a pint of ice cream and binge watch ten hours of *Supernatural*. Seriously. It's a crazy business and we are temperamental artists who can't always wear the armor. Sometimes we like Doritos-stained flannel. But as a producer once told my acting class, "This is the life you chose." And usually I'm pretty darn grateful for it.

Even if I sometimes feel like a dancing monkey magician.

***

Taryn O'Neill is an actress, writer, producer and co-founder of science advocacy group *SCIRENS*. A former competitive figure skater from Vancouver, Canada, and graduate of *Duke University*,

Taryn became an early pioneer in New Media producing the Streamy-nominated sci-fi web series *After Judgment*. She has acted in over 20 web series and such TV shows as *NCIS, Vegas* and *Lie to Me* before being cast as "June Sanders" on BYUTV's 1960's drama *Granite Flats*. As a writer, her first comedy script was a finalist in the NYTVFest FOX Comedy Pilot Contest, she wrote a full length digital series for the incomparable Stan Lee and has numerous web and TV projects in development, sci-fi being her genre of choice. This led to a passion for numerous *STEM* fields, which culminated in the formation of *SCIRENS*, a group of four "sci-enthusiastic" actresses dedicated to using their social media platforms for science outreach and advocacy.

The Downside to Doing What You Love (Followed by the Upside)
By Brea Grant

At the optometrist today, the woman behind the counter asked if she knew me from *Heroes*. I smiled and nodded and normally that experience is far from painful. But today, she asked me that right after I explained to her that I lost my Plan 1 SAG insurance and no longer have my eye care covered. Because I didn't make enough money last year. So not only did I have to explain that somewhat humiliating information, she also knows exactly who I am.

And that is the state I am living in these days. About a year and a half ago, I decided to direct a feature film that I co-wrote and co-starred in. Let me emphasize that it was a great experience and I completely understand what a privilege it is to get to make a movie, much less direct one. I also understand that it is a privilege for me to take time off from my acting career to do something like that. Five years ago, when I was waiting tables, I wouldn't have had the time, money or energy to be able to do that. And although I feel as though I'm having to dust off my acting career and remind everyone that I still exist—because I am finally showing my face some place besides an editing bay—I feel lucky to have a career to dust off in the first place.

So when Helenna asked me to write this piece, which I was stoked on doing, I started with a "dos and don'ts for first time directors," then scratched it for just a blog post about getting distribution for indie films. Then I scratched that and decided to look the metaphorical optometrist woman directly in the eye by facing my (and probably your) fears by writing about doing what I love.

So here is a list of the downsides to doing what you love—a list to read before you start to prepare to write your own screenplay, start a web series, and pursue acting full-time or any project you are driven to do.

1) At the end of the day, you have to care the most.

And that's all you can expect. Yes, your producers should jump up and down when you get into a festival. And yes, your sound person should take pride in getting the very best audio for the project. But for some people, it'll just be a job, and that's okay. Your make-up artist may not want to work three hours into her overtime without pay. It's not her passion project. That can't hurt your feelings. Or even if you are just pursuing an artistic career, at some point, your roommates don't really want to see your audition again or hear that song you've been working on. No one does. But you have to keep working on it.

When it comes to the overall big end product, you have to be the one who sits with it. You have to be the one who wakes up every night for a year thinking you forgot something (or waking up with a moment of genius). You have to give up your weeknights and weekends to do crap that no one else wants to do. And on days when you want to just sleep in or take a break or give up, you can't. Because you are the person who has to give a shit when no one else does.

2) Get ready to give some things up.

Obviously not everyone has to give up his or her health insurance, but you may want to think ahead of time what it is you might have to give up. When I started my movie, my boyfriend at the time said I'd have to give up my acting career to work on it. I scoffed, and while I didn't formally quit acting, I wasn't able to do as well as I did at one time. Think trying to make auditions during pilot season while driving back and forth from my editing bay or turning down movies, particularly in the last few months, because I just didn't have the time. (Now that I think of it, I kind of ended up giving up that boyfriend too.)

So from personal relationships to money to other career aspirations to "me" time, all of it will suffer.

3) Failure is always an option.

Yep. It's the one thing people don't talk about very much. Your movie may not sell. Your web series may not be seen by anyone. Your Kickstarter project may not meet its goal. And you totally talked about it publicly and now everyone knows you're a failure. Or, if you're like me, you don't live up to your giant huge dreams of becoming the next Lena Dunham. I was hoping we'd sell my movie at Slamdance Film Festival for tons of money but we didn't. We signed a distribution contract, but for me that just meant more work, more self-promotion, more of this fucking movie that I've seen four billion times. So, get ready: you take a risk and you can fail. You may not meet your lofty goals. You may not even come close.

Ok. Enough negativity because, for better or for worse, I am a reluctant optimist. Doing what you love means you got to do what you love. You did whatever it is that drives you and not that many people on the planet can say that. You did it. So that's step one.

Let me give you some encouraging words now that I've almost convinced you not to pursue your dreams. You may notice a similarity in these lists.

1) At the end of the day, you probably do care the most.

That is your baby. And you can finish it and say to yourself, "That's my baby" and actually feel really good about it. Or if you didn't finish it, you can say, "At least I tried" because that's more than most people do. Most people just dream. You did far far more.

We just had a cast and crew screening of *Best Friends Forever*, and the nice thing about being a director is that everyone there knows that you work on the movie every day (still…even today). And at the screening, people come up and say nice things to you. Honestly, I don't care if they liked it or are lying about liking it. It just meant a lot that so many people came out to support the movie. It meant the most that people who were a part of the movie came out to support it because it means it wasn't a totally terrible experience for them. They don't completely hate me for not doing what they asked, for leaving their name off the billing block, or for yelling at them on set. I keep replaying that night in my head when I have to answer the 40th email about something I don't care about or as I try to come up with new and creative ways to publicize the movie. Because other people's encouragement means the world. So all that hard work definitely paid off, even in ways I didn't expect it to.

2) Get ready to give things up.

When you have a big change, you sort of get to reevaluate your life. Maybe that guy wasn't really the right guy for you because he didn't support your massive undertaking when you made your own web series. Maybe that day job was shitty and didn't give you the time you needed to get stuff done. Change is hard, but it's a good thing. You're starting something new because you like change. You're pursuing your dreams and doing what you love because it's worth more than anything else. It has to be. Otherwise, you'd still be doing whatever it was you were doing in high school.

3) Failure is always an option.

But the good news is you wouldn't be thinking of doing something like doing what you love if you were scared of failure. You, like me, are the kind of person who likes a risk, who will claw her way to the top, and will stop at nothing to get things done. You don't wait around for people to hand you a career. You are motivated and talented and fuck the world for telling you that you're anything but those things. And you will fail. But the only reason you fail is so you can see how close you were, get back, dust yourself off and try again.

(See what I did there???)

***

Brea Grant is an actress best known for her roles on the hit NBC series *Heroes*, the Showtime original series *Dexter*, and Rob Zombie's *Halloween 2*. She more recently directed the film *Best Friends Forever*, which premiered at Slamdance to great reviews. She is also the creator, writer and co-star of the Nerdist comedy series, *The Real Housewives of Horror*. If you need her, she can generally be found baking vegan cookies or spending time with her dog, Hattie.

Don't Let "The Biz" Get You Down
By Helenna Santos

A little while ago, I found myself having a number of conversations with people in the business about stamina. Basically, the entertainment industry is all about staying focused on "the goal", especially when that goal seems very, very far away, perhaps in another galaxy. There are so many things that can happen to someone pursing a career in this field: exhaustion, disappointment, general malaise with where one is in their career, life feeling like it's taking you in another direction entirely but you aren't sure which path to follow…

In order to thrive and keep putting one foot in front of the other, it's all about always coming at things with a renewed focus and energy, and recommitting oneself every single day.

I asked a number of my friends in "the biz" how they stay motivated when they feel like the industry is conspiring against them. Below are some of the great responses I received:

Dani Lennon: *"I have on many occasions felt this way. The turning point for me was to remember that I LOVE what I do. It's frustrating, but I love it. I remember to continue to have faith and that I put out what I get back. Blah, blah, blah very cliché positive universe crap, but it does help me get back on track. Trying to be positive is a daily struggle but I do find that when I am throwing positive vibes out there I get auditions, interviews and bookings. Keep on fighting! It's worth it. You know making your own projects and producing them gives you that power, channeling that amazing CEO quality. As for the clock ticking, I figured there are nannies, my mother in law to help with the children when life gets busy with auditions and filming. There are trainers to whip my butt into filming shape."*

Jackie Fogel: *"For me, at the point in my life and in my career 'recommitting' each day usually involves me working out in some way. When I'm struggling through some difficult exercise, it reminds me of the challenges in my life and I feel motivated because, difficult or not, I'm doing it. Even on the days where all I do is take a walk, I take time to reflect and check in with myself."*

Amber Plaster: *"I have definitely accomplished a lot this year (especially in the producing world)—and I have to admit I don't have an accountability partner. I never really felt the need for one, as I check in with myself daily, if not hourly. I know that sounds extravagant, but it's true. You should see my notepad on my iPhone. I also use workflowy.com to help my research and complete my daily, monthly and yearly goals. If it gets too overwhelming, I give myself 24 hours to get away from it, feel sorry for myself, complain, or go to the beach, whatever I need to do, then the next morning I attack the to do list with a new fire. I am fortunate enough to have created a day job that I love so I don't hate life every day like I did when I was working at a five star hotel. Maybe it's a first-born child thing? I just figure out three to six things to take care of, sort them in priority, do the smallest thing first, and then reward myself for completing all six tasks. If I have a monthly goal that doesn't get completed, it becomes a daily goal the following month until it gets done. My first quarter was shaky and more unfocused, but by the end of the year, I know exactly what I need more of."*

AJ Meijer: *"Step 1: Get connected with your vision.*
What is it that you want? In the next week? Month? Year? For your life?

Step 2: Write it all down in the form of declaration.
(e.g., I am committed to revamping my actor website by November 1st)

Step 3: Wake up EVERY SINGLE DAY and commit to what you will create that day. (e.g., I commit to going to the gym by 11AM and reading a script by 3PM)
Making it happen will also strengthen your relationship with your word. Which will in turn increase the likelihood of sticking to your commitments. I find reconnecting to my vision so powerful. THAT is what motivates me.

And if for some reason that's not working… the other amazing tool is to "FOCUS OUT". If you need to be inspired, reminded why you're here, reminded why you're doing the things you're doing… give it away, be generous, focus out on others instead of yourself. Volunteer, call a family member or friend you haven't spoken with in a while, create something beautiful for someone and give it away, smile at strangers, the list goes on and on."

For me, I've found that it's all about keeping my eye on the horizon and putting one foot forward and then the other. Sometimes the path is simple and clear, and other times I can barely see the horizon for the trees, but I know it's there. And after all, it's all about the journey. Sometimes even though those trees seem to be in my way, mean and laughing at me with a sadistic grin, they are actually a fun labyrinth-esque obstacle keeping me on my toes, making me appreciate the odyssey that much more.

***

Helenna Santos is an actor, producer, writer, and the founder of *Ms. In The Biz.* She has appeared in a wide variety of projects from feature films such as Universal's *American Reunion*, to high profile digital productions like *BlackBoxTV*, as well as a number of network television series. Helenna can often be found on panels and in appearances at conventions such as San Diego Comic-Con. She has produced and starred in numerous projects including the short horror film *The Infected*, the digital series *Henchmen*, an LGBT experimental short film, and at the time of publishing is in development for the sci-fi creature feature *Specious* and the neo-noir caper flick *Snatched*, both of which she is producing with her husband Barry W. Levy through *Mighty Pharaoh Films.*

PART SIX: Recharge and Take Charge

I Took A Break From Hollywood to Control the "Crazy"
By Deborah Smith

You have heard it time and time again. To be an actor, you must be crazy. Crazy to pursue a dream that is so unscheduled, unorganized, and uncharted. There is no path, and the sheer creative nature of the business makes the journey entirely unique to you.

That right there is the secret to staying sane: this journey is organized, scheduled and charted by YOU. Of course, there is a huge community of people that you should connect with and collaborate with, but here is the one thing you haven't heard: **YOU can control the crazy.**

Let's rewind. I, like most of you out there, fell in love with performing at a very young age. I was a drama geek in junior high and high school. Somewhere along the way, my logical brain kicked in and I decided to do a "safe" major for college. I chose English with a minor in Theater. Laughing at me now? English is basically Theater's second cousin and didn't exactly lead to a high paying job. For many years I was dancing around what I actually wanted to do, act, but fear kept me away. Not fear of failure, but fear of insecurity. **Insecurity was my crazy.**

I have enormous amounts of respect for many of my friends and colleagues who moved to Los Angeles without a dime in their pocket. We have all heard the stories about the actors who slept in their cars so they could pay for acting classes. I knew that I could never be that person. I have experienced financial struggles and knew that I could not be in that space and be creative at the same time. I accepted that, and decided to take a break to control the crazy. I decided to put my dreams in my shirt pocket and earn some savings; that way when I took that dream out, there would be nothing stopping me.

What is your "crazy"? It is extremely important to know your limits in this business. Whether that is nudity, eating ramen noodles every night for dinner or being unable to travel home for the holidays. There is no wrong answer. You must know what will break you, because only when you accept that breaking point can you overcome it.

To overcome my crazy, I became my own business. I am currently working on web design, marketing and copywriting for five clients in the US and Australia. I make my own hours, set my own schedule and chart my own journey. Best of all, I have harnessed the insecurity and now use it to my advantage. Hollywood is a business, and I am using my skills as a businesswoman to make my mark.

Of course, being an entrepreneur has its challenges, but it also has immense benefits. Yes, I am older than most actresses "starting out", but I also have life experience that benefits my art, knowledge of the world outside of Hollywood, and a passion that has been burning for the last 15 years. For the first time in my life, I have taken my dreams out of my pocket and put them in my hand.

Think about what is holding you back from success. What is your "crazy"? Maybe you need to accept your crazy and learn how to harness it to benefit you. You can be your greatest asset and biggest competition. There are a lot of other people out there fighting for the same role. You don't want to be in your own way. Learn to control the crazy, and take a break if you need to. Believe me, you will come back more tenacious, dedicated and passionate than you would have ever thought possible.

***

Deborah Smith is an actress and entrepreneur whose love of performing, learning and new experiences has led to travels around the globe. Originally from LA, she studied at *UC Berkeley* before moving to Australia to pursue her Master's degree in Film Production & Marketing. She worked in the Australian film industry while starting her own marketing/web design freelance business and has now returned to Los Angeles to chase her dream of becoming the girl-next-door turned unlikely superhero. She loves developing characters and writing about powerful historical figures whose tales go unheard!

Press Play: Check in With Your Inner Artist (In Private)
By Taryn O'Neill

You get up, check your email, your news feed, Twitter, you tweet something, links, feelings, comments, your meditation, you run to the gym, your day job, juggling five projects you're working on, on the side, in your head, writing while you write, thinking while you think, multiple levels of processing going on as you blog, video blog, network, always on, always connected. Coffee, drinks, meet ups—everything is live, in the now—

Your creativity is running a triathlon. Full steam ahead, focused, ambitious, purposeful. Because we are always "on", connected, even when we are at play—on vacation, at a convention or a meet up. And it's not that we aren't also exercising our soul: we live in a state of inspiration, a TED Talk or a Tiny Buddha in every corner. We read it, revel in it, then share it! It's not just enough to read it, think about it ourselves and then let it go. There are tiny cute buttons at the bottom of the article that beg for you to share.

Does this ring a bell?

I thought it might. Now, Breathe.

I believe there is no time dedicated to developing our art, our soul, in private. There is this pressure that we're always discovering and creating in public, even if we're taking a break. Everything is an Instagram, maybe a latergram, but never a nevergram. Why would we process and build without a public's opinion?

I think as busy multi-hyphenate women, we need that reprise, that recharge, where nothing is at stake or being judged. With being connected, you are always present for "feedback". Others are shaping your ideas and your work, even if you don't realize it.

I have been reading *The Artist's Way* again and am enrolled in Tara Mohr's *Playing Big*. Both stress the importance of The Artist Date and taking time to nurture your inner artist/inner child. I then stumbled on a great *TED Talk* (of course) on the subject of play and the lack of it in adult lives. As many of us work in entertainment, however, there is a certain amount of "play" that goes along with the work that we do. It's entertainment after all, but I realized that even when we think we are "playing", we are live-blogging it, commenting on it in our various social platforms. It's become "play as a contest". So how can we break free and regain the innocence of truly playing?

I've come up with a few suggestions that I'm hoping to follow:

1) Make a pact with yourself <u>that you are enough</u>.
You don't need the approval of your family, friends or social networks. Repeat that again: you don't need the approval of your family, friends or social networks.

2) Put away your connected devices for a set amount of time.
An hour a day? A weekend? One day a month? If you can't do that, at least hide your social network apps in a folder on your fourth screen. And name the folder "Taxes" or "Accounting" or "Sit ups".

3) There are articles, posts, books and videos you probably want to watch as part of your artist date in order to recharge. But create space away from the connected screen.
Treat them like you would your favorite hardcover book. Have a notebook with you to jot down notes and thoughts that these articles inspire.

4) Plan outings that we can call Play Dates.
These are activities where you really get to PLAY. No judgment from the outside world, a date that you take with your inner artist child that is just your own—no one else's—where you can savor an experience on your own.

Here are some ideas of **Play Dates** that I've come up with:

1) The Best Field Trip Ever.

Remember what it was like when you went on a field trip? When you got to go on a bus with your friends heading to some quasi-educational but quasi-fun location? You got to get out of math and biology! You probably got to eat a different type of lunch, you probably got in trouble for not staying with the group, but you definitely had fun... and I bet you were "awed" by something you saw. Not that you would admit it.

So let's do that... Where did you go? The aquarium, the zoo, the circus, the planetarium, the observatory... Plan an afternoon there, save the ticket stubs. Have your school notebook and make notes, or just write a note to the cute guy across the food court.

2) The Moody Road Trip.

Embrace your inner Jack Kerouac or Hunter S Thompson. Take a road trip to somewhere you've wanted to go, equipped with only your notebook and maybe a disposable camera, and see what stories you stumble upon. Be open to the beauty. Be open to connection. And then take the time and the privacy to see what you captured, what the pieces suggest, maybe they exist as separate moments, but maybe there is a larger narrative. Sketch, write, remember: see how jotting down the memory of something that happened as opposed to transcribing it. Wait for the film to be developed.

3) The Terribly Terrible Awesome Play.

Remember when you acted in your first play in kindergarten—how awful and wonderful it was all at once? This was probably the first time you ever stepped onto a stage in someone else's shoes. And you were probably awful. But I bet you loved every minute of it. The sheer craziness of having no idea what you were doing. The play was the thing. This is what we are talking about after all, right? The Play? Playing? How the term "player" got twisted into a negative image is unfortunate. But let's return to the origins of the word—which is movement, to leap, jump. My old acting teacher said that the best thing you could do for yourself as an actor was to direct something.

By doing that, you are breaking out of the norm, breaking gravity—you are leaping. So do something you are not good at: paint, write, create, shoot, sing, dance, as long as it is not good! Good is the enemy! Be bad and embrace it, like when you were young… but what does bad mean to you? Bad could be great. Or it could just be bad, but it will shed light on something.

4) A Secret Date with your Inner Mentor.

Who do you revere? Whose work inspires you, motivates you, guides you internally? If you happened to have a day with them, where would you go? What areas of your city would you want them to take you to because they could shed new light on something? What areas would you never go if not for their presence? Bring along a book or an interview on them that you can read while you are out on your date. Use their work and your imagination to step into their shoes. Be inspired but also brought to awareness through their humanity. Their journey might not have been so different than yours. (And just as if you were out with a celebrity, tweeting your adventures would not be encouraged.)

There are countless creative things you can do to have play dates. One of my favorite finds is *ForYourArt.com*—an email feed that aggregates all the "art" going on in your city that weekend. But being cultured and inspired shouldn't be a competitive sport that is judged by the number of Instagram likes it has. Fight the desire to have others comment on your experience. Just one time. Easier said than done, right? But I'm looking forward to seeing how it feels.

Your private play should be experienced, savored, reflected on. Not judged. Just keep playing.

***

Taryn O'Neill is an actress, writer, producer and co-founder of science advocacy group *SCIRENS*. A former competitive figure skater from Vancouver, Canada, and graduate of *Duke University*, Taryn became an early pioneer in New Media producing the Streamy-nominated sci-fi web series *After Judgment*. She has acted in over 20 web series and such TV shows as *NCIS, Vegas* and *Lie to Me* before being cast as "June Sanders" on BYUTV's 1960's drama *Granite Flats*. As a writer, her first comedy script was a finalist in the *NYTVFest FOX* Comedy Pilot Contest, she wrote a full length digital series for the incomparable Stan Lee and has numerous web and TV projects in development, sci-fi being her genre of choice. This led to a passion for numerous *STEM* fields, which culminated in the formation of *SCIRENS*, a group of four 'sci-enthusiastic' actresses dedicated to using their social media platforms for science outreach and advocacy.

How to Get Luckier
By Samara Bay

"She's so lucky."

We've all thought it. A dash of vinegar, before we quickly attempt to turn it sweet. But I'm not here to talk about the abundance principle—that there's enough to go around and a win for one member of our field is a win for all. I mean, I'm a big proponent of that philosophy, 'cuz life is totally better if we believe it. But I'm not talking about it. I'm talking about:

What if *we* were the lucky ones that evoked the response above?

Maybe you think of yourself as lucky already—God knows, we all work on gratitude in this town. But do you twinkle with just a little more sense of good fortune than your friends? Do good things just seem to follow you around? Are you on a winning streak? Was there that one chance connection that led to that thing that led to that other thing that led to the job you have now, which is awesome? All of us could probably answer yes to the above—but perhaps a bit half-heartedly: "Yeah, I guess I'm lucky… but I mean… I could be more so, if that's what you're asking."

My mom recently sent me a link to one of those Articles That Make You Think. One that, as it turns out, was more than a decade old, but it totally stands the test of time: in it a psychology professor convincingly, and rather charmingly, argues that luck can be learned. By anyone. As long as there's a little more intuition at play, some breaking-up of the ol' routine, and perhaps a tad more goofy optimism in the mix.

Sounds like a perfect recipe for us crazy industry folk.

The professor, Dr. Richard Wiseman of the University of Hertfordshire, describes collecting hundreds of test subjects, unassuming Englishmen and women of all ages who self-identified as either lucky or unlucky people, and then spending years asking them to participate in various experiments and submit diary entries and answer questionnaires and take personality tests. And some very noticeable trends began to appear: although no one quite knew *why* they were lucky, their behaviors and thought patterns totally gave it away.

This experiment says it best. The professor writes:

I gave both lucky and unlucky people a newspaper, and asked them to look through it and tell me how many photographs were inside. On average, the unlucky people took about two minutes to count the photographs, whereas the lucky people took just seconds. Why? Because the second page of the newspaper contained the message: "Stop counting. There are 43 photographs in this newspaper." This message took up half of the page and was written in type that was more than 2 inches high. It was staring everyone straight in the face, but the unlucky people tended to miss it and the lucky people tended to spot it.

For fun, I placed a second large message halfway through the newspaper: "Stop counting. Tell the experimenter you have seen this and win £250." Again, the unlucky people missed the opportunity because they were still too busy looking for photographs.

This is the thing. We can go through life wondering why it's so much more difficult for us to get what we want than it is for others despite working sooooo hard (bless Facebook for compounding that particular neurosis), or we can stop focusing so much on getting what we want... and end up actually getting it. Not necessarily because focus itself is bad or because life is a cosmic joke. Rather because the act of relaxing around a goal frees us up to achieve it in UNEXPECTED WAYS. Focus is fine; tension is icky. (For anyone who's read *The Artist's Way*: synchronicity!) According to Dr. Wiseman, "personality tests revealed that unlucky people are generally much more tense than lucky people, and research has shown that anxiety disrupts people's ability to notice the unexpected [...] Unlucky people miss chance opportunities because they are too focused on looking for something else."

If we go to a networking event hoping to find someone useful for our career, we'll probably feel gross and also, relatedly, fail. So there's that. But if we go open to connecting with awesome new people, we may very well find someone useful for our career by accident, or someone who leads to someone who leads to someone. Or the love of our life. Or none of the above, but a renewed sense of confidence and social ease, which will likely help with those other goals down the line.

Clichéd but true: it can't hurt to try.

So I say, here's to going home a different way and lingering to chat with that interesting person and saying "yes" to random outings or events despite a flutter of anxiety. 'Cuz comfort zones are for the unlucky. Here's to taking comfort instead in the new—in surreal, magical, unexpected treats we may never have found in that musty old zone. Turns out, when Dr. Wiseman suggested to his "unlucky" group that they spend a month following some prompts that would help them do more of what the "lucky" folks did, there was an 80 percent uptick in happiness and satisfaction. And what were those prompts?

- Make decisions more intuitively—think, yes, but feel too. Follow hunches. Your gut knows.
- Introduce more variety into your life. Not only go to events you might not otherwise have attended, but also talk to everyone there wearing red. Or sparkles. Or of the mustachioed persuasion. Make up games for yourself. Randomness breeds luck.
- *Expect* good stuff to find you. There is, of course, this self-fulfilling thing about life, eh? Eeyores will be Eeyores, until they decide not to be.
- Remember, it could have been worse. In Dr. Wiseman's interviews the "lucky" people would tell stories of crappy situations they'd been in—situations of equal crappiness to the "unlucky" people's tales of woe, in fact—but somehow

these lucky folks would see the bright side instead. So pull a little *Silver Linings Playbook* on that crap.

Tellingly, when pressed by a *Fast Company* interviewer with "but can we acknowledge that sometimes bad stuff—car accidents, natural disasters—just happens? Sometimes it's purely bad, and there's nothing good about it," how did the good doctor respond?

"I've never heard that from a lucky person."

***

Samara Bay is a dialect and communication coach for actors, hosts and members of the science, tech and business arenas. She writes about the intersection of creative culture and innovation, moderates panels at Silicon Beach conferences, and was on the leadership council of the UN's first ever summit on media for social impact. She's an Ambassador of co-working space *WeWork*, an Advocate for *artworxLA*, an Al Gore-trained *Climate Reality Leader*, and a member of the *Alan Alda Center for Communicating Science*. Recent films Samara has dialect coached include *Captain America: The Winter Soldier*, *X-MEN: Days of Future Past,* and Kevin Smith's *Yoga Hosers.*

Conclusion

So here we are.

As our colleagues over at the *Inside Acting Podcast* say, whether "you feel this career and life chose you, or you chose it," you have made a commitment to the creative, and you are taking the steps to kick some serious industry butt!

So go for it! Not just in a half-baked way. But REALLY go for it.

Arm yourself with knowledge. Rest when you need to rest, push on when you need to push on. Share what you've learned with others because we all rise to the top together. Find your tribe. Be tenacious. Be helpful. Be loving. Be kind. And most importantly, be YOU. There is only one of you, and this industry needs to know the authentic you that is so special and so unique because what you bring to the biz is more valuable than you realize. So show your artistic heart, expand your business savvy brain, and we'll see you in that glorious space between action and cut where everything and anything is possible.

- Helenna and Alexandra

Join the Ms. In The Biz Community!

Interested in becoming involved with the *Ms. In The Biz* Community? Head on over to **msinthebiz.com** and sign up for updates on events, articles, and more! If you are a female entertainment industry professional and would like to write for *Ms. In The Biz*, feel free to reach out to us via our "contact" page on the site.

We can also be found on Twitter at: **twitter.com/msinthebiz** and on Facebook at: **facebook.com/msinthebiz**

About Helenna Santos

Helenna Santos is an actor, producer, writer, and the founder of *Ms. In The Biz*. She has appeared in a wide variety of projects from feature films such as Universal's *American Reunion*, to high profile digital productions like *BlackBoxTV*, as well as a number of network television series. Helenna can often be found on panels and in appearances at conventions such as San Diego Comic-Con. She has produced and starred in numerous projects including the short horror film *The Infected*, the digital series *Henchmen*, an LGBT experimental short film, and at the time of publishing is in development for the sci-fi creature feature *Specious* and the neo-noir caper flick *Snatched*, both of which she is producing with her husband Barry W. Levy through *Mighty Pharaoh Films*.

About Alexandra Boylan

Alexandra Boylan was born and raised in Georgetown, Massachusetts, where she first began her exploration into acting, which led her to relocate to Los Angeles. After working in the industry, she soon realized her true calling as a producer. She co-founded *MirrorTree Productions* which has produced two feature films, *Home Sweet Home* and *Catching Faith*. Alexandra is also the Co-Creator of *Your Perfect Adventure* which just released the first of its kind live action, movie, app game, *Your Pizza Adventure,* which brings a new platform of entertainment to the world, melding video games and movies into one. She is an active member of *Women in Film* in Los Angeles and hopes to continue to create strong female-driven content for audiences everywhere.

Made in the USA
San Bernardino, CA
27 December 2014